ADVANCES IN HEALTH AND DISEASE

ADVANCES IN HEALTH AND DISEASE

VOLUME 3

ADVANCES IN HEALTH AND DISEASE

Additional books in this series can be found on Nova's website under the Series tab.

Additional e-books in this series can be found on Nova's website under the eBooks tab.

ADVANCES IN HEALTH AND DISEASE

ADVANCES IN HEALTH AND DISEASE

VOLUME 3

LOWELL T. DUNCAN
EDITOR

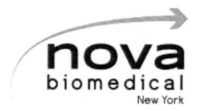

Copyright © 2018 by Nova Science Publishers, Inc.

All rights reserved. No part of this book may be reproduced, stored in a retrieval system or transmitted in any form or by any means: electronic, electrostatic, magnetic, tape, mechanical photocopying, recording or otherwise without the written permission of the Publisher.

We have partnered with Copyright Clearance Center to make it easy for you to obtain permissions to reuse content from this publication. Simply navigate to this publication's page on Nova's website and locate the "Get Permission" button below the title description. This button is linked directly to the title's permission page on copyright.com. Alternatively, you can visit copyright.com and search by title, ISBN, or ISSN.

For further questions about using the service on copyright.com, please contact:
Copyright Clearance Center
Phone: +1-(978) 750-8400   Fax: +1-(978) 750-4470   E-mail: info@copyright.com.

NOTICE TO THE READER

The Publisher has taken reasonable care in the preparation of this book, but makes no expressed or implied warranty of any kind and assumes no responsibility for any errors or omissions. No liability is assumed for incidental or consequential damages in connection with or arising out of information contained in this book. The Publisher shall not be liable for any special, consequential, or exemplary damages resulting, in whole or in part, from the readers' use of, or reliance upon, this material. Any parts of this book based on government reports are so indicated and copyright is claimed for those parts to the extent applicable to compilations of such works.

Independent verification should be sought for any data, advice or recommendations contained in this book. In addition, no responsibility is assumed by the publisher for any injury and/or damage to persons or property arising from any methods, products, instructions, ideas or otherwise contained in this publication.

This publication is designed to provide accurate and authoritative information with regard to the subject matter covered herein. It is sold with the clear understanding that the Publisher is not engaged in rendering legal or any other professional services. If legal or any other expert assistance is required, the services of a competent person should be sought. FROM A DECLARATION OF PARTICIPANTS JOINTLY ADOPTED BY A COMMITTEE OF THE AMERICAN BAR ASSOCIATION AND A COMMITTEE OF PUBLISHERS.

Additional color graphics may be available in the e-book version of this book.

Library of Congress Cataloging-in-Publication Data

ISBN: 978-1-53613-020-1

Published by Nova Science Publishers, Inc. † New York

CONTENTS

Preface vii

Chapter 1 Neuroendocrine Regulation of
Homeostasis in Insects:
Implications for Metabolic Disorders in Humans 1
*Andrea Bednářová, Dalibor Kodrík,
Anathbandhu Chaudhuri and Natraj Krishnan*

Chapter 2 Exploring Micro -, Mezzo -, and Macro- Level
Factors Impacting HIV Testing Behaviors among
Asian Americans and Pacific Islander 47
*Soma Sen, Van Ta Park, Malaya Arevalo,
So Yung Kim and Hoang Dung Nguyen*

Chapter 3 Removing Heteroplasmic Mitochondrial
DNA Mutations 83
*Juan M. Suárez-Rivero, Marina Villanueva-Paz,
Suleva Povea-Cabello, Mario de la Mata,
Irene Villalón-García, Mónica Álvarez-Córdoba,
David Cotán and José A. Sánchez-Alcázar*

Chapter 4	The Attachment and Its Role in Medical Care *Carlo Lai, Gaia Romana Pellicano,* *Daniela Altavilla, Laura Pierro, Erika Fazzari,* *Edvaldo Begotaraj, Giada Lucarelli, Paola Aceto* *and Massimiliano Luciani*	**119**
Chapter 5	Hip Dislocation: Types, Causes and Treatments *Alessandro Aprato, Michele Nardi, Marco Favuto,* *Gabriele Cominetti, Kristijan Zoccola* *and Alessandro Massè*	**149**
Chapter 6	Multicentric Castleman Disease: Associated and Differential Disorders *Yoshinori Tanino and Hiroyuki Minemura*	**173**
Chapter 7	Influence of Gut Microbiota on Inflammatory Bowel Disease *Dennis Cesar Levano-Linares,* *Patricia Sanchez-Salcedo, David Alias-Jimenez,* *Belen Manso-Abajo, Ana Moreno-Posada* *and Jaime Ruiz-Tovar*	**197**
Chapter 8	Sudden Death *Luca Roncati, Antonio Manenti* *and Giuseppe Barbolini*	**217**
Chapter 9	Amantadine for Parkinson's Disease *Shaheen E. Lakhan and Muhammad Safwatullah*	**229**
Index		**237**

Preface

In this compilation, the authors begin by examining the correlation between stress tolerance, metabolism, and energy balance using insects as model systems and demonstrate how in recent years, the authors have learned mostly from physiological responses in insects that many parallels exist between invertebrate and mammalian homeostasis. Therefore, studying insects as simpler model organisms can provide useful information for elucidating the complexities of mammalian metabolism. Following this, the book presents a mixed-methods study with the goal of adding to the existing body of knowledge in the areas of HIV-related risk behaviors, HIV testing behaviors, and the various factors that act as barriers and facilitators to HIV testing among Asian Americans and Pacific Islanders. The authors go on to deliberate on the advantages and disadvantages of potential strategies for the treatment of mitochondrial diseases caused by mutant mtDNA. As cells contain multiple copies of mtDNA, pathogenic mtDNA mutations frequently coexist with wild-type mtDNA, a phenomenon known as "heteroplasmy". The patient attachment style is investigated as a moderator of the patient and practitioner relationship in order to potentially promote clinical interventions aimed to enhance the adherence to medical care, improving health-care outcomes and patient quality of life. Next, the patterns of dislocation and subluxation are reviewed, along with associated issues, in order to allow surgeons to provide optimal care for these patients. Hip dislocation or subluxation may occur after surgical procedure and has been reported after hip arthroscopy and other open procedures. The authors discuss Castleman's disease, a rare lymphoproliferative syndrome derived into two groups: unicentric and multicentric. Unicentric Castleman's disease is presented as an isolated mass, such as mediastitial lymph node, and is curable with surgery in most cases. Multicentric Castleman's diseaseis comprised of heterogeneous disorders with various etiologies and represents systemic inflammatory symptoms, such as fever and weight loss. The subsequent chapter discusses the evidence concerning the involvement of microbiota on the appearance and development of inflammatory bowel diseases and the eventual response to medical treatment. Despite promising links between microbial composition and disease phenotypes, to date no causative role for the microbiome has been established, and our understanding of the dynamic role of the human microbiome in inflammatory bowel diseases remains incomplete. The book also examines sudden death, an unexpected event that happens in healthy people or in stable patients. It must occur within one hour from the onset of the first symptoms, and it is precipitated by a cardiac arrest, which is irreversible due to the absence of adequate assistance. In closing, amantadine is examined in the context of treatment of Parkinson's disease and its complications. As a tricyclic amine, it enhances the release of dopamine at the synaptic cleft and inhibits its uptake, acts directly at the D2 receptor and up-regulates it, has anti-muscarinic properties, and non-competitive antagonism of the NMDA receptor. It has been studied as both a monotherapy or adjuvant therapy for Parkinson's disease with mixed results.

Chapter 1 - The homeostatic environment in an organism is under constant challenge by internal and external stressors. Responding to stress is an energy demanding process and takes a toll on energy balance. Hence, energy homeostasis is a fundamental requirement in an organism's adaptive response to stress. The ability of an organism to tolerate and respond to stress is critical to its establishment and persistence in specific localities. This is particularly so in insects, which have successfully occupied most environmental niches and their continued success depends on responding effectively to and surviving a broad range of environmental stressors including temperature, desiccation, xenobiotic, osmotic and infection stress.

In insects, the behavioral and physiological responses to diverse stressors are coordinated by the actions of various neurotransmitters and (neuro)hormones to facilitate stress induced changes ultimately leading to regulation of energy balance. Though the root cause of the mechanisms responsible for efficient energy homeostasis may remain contested, the central role of the brain in regulating energy balance remains undisputed. It could be argued that the emergence and evolution of the central nervous system is to promote the most effective means of dealing with energy homeostasis. Thus, the perception of stress leads to changes in the secretion profile of specific transmitters/hormones which essentially facilitate the modulation of physiology and behavior. Further, insulin-like peptides (ILPs) and adipokinetic hormones (AKHs) are neuropeptides that have similar roles as mammalian insulin and glucagon, respectively. The neurotransmitter dopamine (DA) has also been implicated in feeding and satiety responses bringing in possibilities of a complex neuro-regulatory network involved in energy homeostasis. These compounds - insulin, glucagon and increasingly also DA are critical components of metabolic pathways that regulate energy homeostasis in mammals. Dysfunctions in energy homeostasis mechanisms result in metabolic disorders such as obesity and diabetes in humans which represent a major public health challenge around the world. The authors explored the links between stress tolerance, metabolism, and energy balance using insects as model systems and demonstrate how in recent years, they have learned mostly from physiological responses in insects that many parallels exist between invertebrate and mammalian homeostasis. Thus, investigations on insects as simpler model organisms can provide useful information for elucidating the complexities of mammalian metabolism. An increased understanding of neural circuits underlying control of energy homeostasis is key for development of novel therapies in treatment of obesity and associated co-morbidities, including diabetes.

Chapter 2 - Asian Americans and Pacific Islanders (AAPI) are the only racial group in the U.S. with a significant increase in HIV rates and delayed HIV testing. However, factors impacting HIV testing in this population is poorly understood. Hence, this mixed method study examines the various individual, familial, structural factors that impact testing behavior in this population. Findings revealed various barriers to testing including a lack of HIV related knowledge and low perception of risk, a family culture of silence around HIV, HIV related stigma, fear of losing social/sexual networks, and fear of dealing with the diagnosis alone. These findings indicate a necessity to understand the decision making process that impact HIV testing and to design interventions to mitigate the impact of stigma.

Chapter 3 - Mitochondrial diseases are inborn error disorders caused by total or partial dysfunction of the mitochondrial respiratory chain. These disorders are associated with a wide variety of metabolic and systemic diseases affecting the brain, muscle, heart, retina, optic nerve, liver and endocrine organs. Although many mitochondrial diseases are caused by mutations in the nuclear DNA (nDNA), some of them are due to mutations in the mitochondrial DNA (mtDNA). As cells contain multiple copies of mtDNA, pathogenic mtDNA mutations frequently coexist with wild-type mtDNA, a phenomenon termed heteroplasmy. Disease phenotypes are only observed once the proportion of wild-type mtDNA drops below a threshold level associated with high accumulations of heteroplasmic mutations. Generally, a critical threshold level above 60-80% of heteroplasmy is required to trigger the oxidative phosphorylation (OXPHOS) defects in specific tissues. Therefore, increasing the proportion of wild-type mtDNA in affected tissues is seen as a viable therapeutic strategy for the treatment of diseases caused by mtDNA mutations.

Nowadays, several heteroplasmy removal/reduction strategies have been proposed (Figure 1). The pharmacologic approach with rapamycin (an autophagy activator) treatment has shown promising results in transmitochondrial cybrid cell lines. Heteroplasmy reduction has been also achieved by the overexpression of mitophagy related proteins such as Parkin. Finally, genome editing via endonucleases, transcription activator-like effector nucleases (TALENs), zinc finger nucleases (ZFNs) and clustered regularly interspaced short palindromic repeats (CRISPR) system represent novel and efficient approaches to treat mitochondrial pathologies in cell models. In this chapter, the authors will discuss about the advantages and disadvantages of these potential strategies for the treatment of mitochondrial diseases caused by mutant mtDNA.

Chapter 4 - Attachment styles are relational models that lead an individual to seek proximity to a safe or powerful person when threatened. As suggested by attachment theory, the quality of early interpersonal experiences shapes the self-regulate ability during the entire life span and modulate the complex relationship between social, cognitive, and emotional variables. The attachment system seems to be strongly involved in the health-related events, due to its self-regulation function. Individuals with physical illness are forced to cope with new people, contexts and experiences that are potential stressors of attachment system. Relational models, thus, seem to have a significant role in health-related psychological processes, in particular, on patients' ability to engage in a fruitful alliance with their physicians. Major chronic conditions and their complex management could broadly take advantage from a safely and trustful relationship between patient and physician. Patient medical adherence is a basic statement in health care and recent studies reported that it is closely associated with the affective relationship between patient and practitioner. Investigating the patient attachment style as a moderator of this relationship could promote clinical interventions aimed to enhance the adherence to medical care, improving health-care outcomes and patient quality of life.

Chapter 5 - Hip dislocation or subluxation may appear in a wide range of settings: it may result from traumatic injury, atraumatic capsular laxity, structural bony abnormality (such as acetabular dysplasia) and iatrogenic injury.

Traumatic hip dislocations, most often caused by motor vehicle accidents or similar high-energy impacts, traverse a large subset of distinct injury patterns. Non-surgical treatment is often recommended if no other associated injuries occurred while surgical treatment may be required in selected cases and may be performed arthroscopically or trough open surgery.

Dislocation may also occur after a minor trauma; in those cases often a predisposing anatomy is the leading cause of the instability. Treatment is controversial in those scenarios but surgeon should evaluate the femoral and acetabular anatomy and, if indicated, offer its possible correction such as periacetabular osteotomy and/or femoral osteotomy.

Atraumatic subluxation of the hip is often present in patients with developmental dysplasia of the hip. The latter involves a spectrum of hip disorders that affect hip anatomy and development and can range from mild anatomical deformity with a reduced but subluxable hip to a frankly dislocated hip.

Eventually hip dislocation or subluxation may occur after surgical procedure and they have been reported after either hip arthroscopy either open procedures. In those cases, treatment is controversial and often ends in a total hip replacement.

In this chapter, the patterns of dislocation and subluxation are reviewed and their associated issue are described in order to allow surgeons to provide optimal care for these patients.

Chapter 6 - Castleman's disease (CD) is a rare lymphoproliferative syndrome, and is derived into two groups: unicentric and multicentric. Unicentric Castleman's disease is presented as an isolated mass, such as mediastitial lymph node, and is curable with surgery in most cases. Multicentric Castleman's disease (MCD) is comprised of heterogeneous disorders with various etiologies and represents systemic inflammatory symptoms, such as fever and weight loss. Human herpes virus-8 (HHV-8) is thought to be a causable pathogen in all HIV-positive MCD patients, as well as some HIV-negative MCD patients, via hypercytokinemia. Definitive diagnosis of MCD is difficult because a variety of disorders, such as malignancy, inflammatory and infectious diseases, represent MCD-like features. Recently, the term, idiopathic MCD (iMCD) has been proposed as HHV-8-negative MCD by the international, evidence-based consensus diagnostic criteria. Although the diagnostic criteria requires to exclude various disorders which show similar clinical characteristics as MCD to make a diagnosis of iMCD, it is difficult to differentiate these similar disorders such as malignant lymphoma, autoimmune diseases, POEMS syndrome, IgG4-related disease, autoimmune lymphoproliferative syndrome (ALPS) and virus infection from MCD. In addition, there has been an intense debate on the difference between the disorders and MCD. That is, it has not been clarified if MCD is exactly different from these disorders or is the associated clinical phenotype of them. The authors recently reported a case of MCD with ALPS, which is a rare nonmalignant lymphoproliferative disorder characterized by increase in CD3+TCRαβ+CD4-CD8- double-negative T (DNT) cells and peripheral lymphadenopathy. The authors herein discuss the association and difference between MCD and various disorders that represent MCD-like features.

Chapter 7 - Inflammatory bowel disease (IBD) is a chronic, multifactorial immune disorder and it is classified in two different entities with unknown etiologies: Crohn's Disease and Ulcerative Colitis. However, it is believed that disturbance of the immune system and/or imbalanced interactions with microbes (dysbioses) leads to development of chronic intestinal inflammation. Over the past decade, IBD have emerged as one of the most studied human conditions linked to the gut microbiota. More recently, profiling studies of the intestinal microbiome have associated pathogenesis of IBD with characteristic shifts in the composition of the intestinal microbiota, reinforcing the view that IBD result from altered interactions between intestinal microbes and the mucosal immune system. On the other hand, several pathogens have been proposed as causative microorganisms for IBD development. Several factors can intervene with microbial gut community composition, including genetics, diet, age, drug treatment or smoking. The importance of each of these factors is still unclear, but several of them are directly or indirectly linked to disease state.

Some studies show that the gut microbiota is an essential factor in driving inflammation in IBD and indeed, short-term treatment with some antibiotics reduces intestinal inflammation.

The improvements to DNA sequencing technology have set the stage for investigations of the IBD microbiome. Many studies find dysbioses, that occur in IBD and a broad pattern has begun to emerge which includes a reduction in biodiversity, a decreased and an increased representation of several taxa. As opposed, several lines of evidence suggest that specific groups of gut bacteria may have protective effects against IBD.

It is important to mention that some of the alterations observed in the colorectal cancer (CRC) microbiome are also observed in IBD, and chronic intestinal inflammation is a major risk factor for the development of CRC.

Despite promising correlations between microbial composition and disease phenotypes, to date no causative role for the microbiome has been established, and our understanding of the dynamic role of the human microbiome in IBD remains incomplete.

In this chapter, the authors will discuss the actual evidence about the involvement of microbiota on the appearance and development of IBD, and the eventual response to medical treatment.

Chapter 8 - Sudden death can be defined as an unexpected event that happens in healthy people or in stable patients. It must occur within one hour from the onset of the first symptoms, and it is precipitated by a cardiac arrest, which is irreversible for the absence of an adequate and prompt assistance or for an intrinsic cardiac disease.

Heart block is usually preceded by severe disturbances of the cardiac rhythm, as ventricular fibrillation or bradycardia. In a first group of diseases, at the basis of this event, a primitive disorder, directly correlated with an abnormality of cell membrane channels involved in the exchange of electrolytes, can be found, as in Brugada's syndrome.

A more common condition is represented by infarct or severe ischemia, sometimes known before, that determine significant alterations in the cardiac rhythm, followed by ventricular fibrillation and cardiac arrest.

Rarer is an acute hemopericardium, where a sudden severe haemorrhage takes place inside the pericardium, with a primary effect of acute cardiac tamponade; in absence of recent cardio-thoracic surgery, a cause can be the rupture of an aortic aneurysm, involving its first intrapericardic tract.

Many other cardiac diseases, as acute myocarditis, left ventricular hypertrophy, hypertrophic cardiomyopathy, dilatative cardiomyopathy, restrictive cardiomyopathy, Arrhythmogenic Right Ventricular Cardiomyopathy (ARVC), pulmonary or aortic stenosis, atrial myxoma, and, rarely, Cyanotic Congenital Heart Diseases (CCHD), can induce a sudden cardiac arrest.

In other conditions, the cardiac arrest follows an acute primary disease of one or multiple apparatuses. At first, an abrupt and massive haemorrhage, followed by a fall in the venous return, can produce an electro-mechanical cardiac dissociation, with subsequent cardiac arrest. A similar condition is represented by anaphylactic shock, where a sudden peripheral vasodilatation with an abrupt fall in blood venous return can be associated with an increased pulmonary vascular resistance, bronchospasm and coronary vasoconstriction by circulating histamine. A characteristic condition is the onset of an acute respiratory failure, followed by acute hypoxia, hypercapnia and acidosis. It can happen after tension pneumothorax, complicating a respiratory insufficiency, or in case of bilateral pneumothorax.

Moreover, a sudden increase in pulmonary resistance accompanied by severe hypoxia, as in acute thrombo-embolism of the pulmonary artery, can determine a sudden cardiac arrest. Another cause, even rarer, of cardiac arrest is finally represented by a spontaneous cerebral haemorrhage, where a rapid rise of intracranial pressure, but more often a direct damage of vital cerebral centres, leads to a direct acute cardio-respiratory failure.

Chapter 9 - From a single case use in 1969, amantadine has been shown to be efficacious in the treatment of Parkinson's disease and its complications. As a tricyclic amine, it enhances the release of dopamine at the synaptic cleft and inhibits its uptake, acts directly at the D2 receptor and up-regulates it, has anti-muscarinic properties, and non-competitive antagonism of the NMDA receptor. It has been studied as both a monotherapy or adjuvant therapy for Parkinson's disease with mixed results. Likewise, it has been investigated for other neurodegenerative conditions such as multiple system atrophy, progressive supranuclear palsy, and other akinetic-rigid syndromes. Its long-term effects are being delineated.

In: Advances in Health and Disease
Editor: Lowell T. Duncan

ISBN: 978-1-53613-020-1
© 2018 Nova Science Publishers, Inc.

Chapter 1

NEUROENDOCRINE REGULATION OF HOMEOSTASIS IN INSECTS: IMPLICATIONS FOR METABOLIC DISORDERS IN HUMANS

Andrea Bednářová[1,2,*], *Dalibor Kodrík*[1,3], *Anathbandhu Chaudhuri*[4] *and Natraj Krishnan*[3]

[1]Institute of Entomology, Biology Centre, Academy of Sciences, České Budějovice, Czech Republic
[2]Department of Biochemistry, Molecular Biology, Entomology and Plant Pathology, Mississippi State University, MS, US
[3]Faculty of Science, University of South Bohemia, České Budějovice, Czech Republic
[4]Department of Natural Sciences, Stinson Mathematics and Science Building, 3601 Stillman Blvd, Stillman College, Tuscaloosa, AL, US

---

[*]Corresponding Author E-mail: a.bednarova@entu.cas.cz; Phone: +420-387 775 265; Fax: +420 385 310 354.

ABSTRACT

The homeostatic environment in an organism is under constant challenge by internal and external stressors. Responding to stress is an energy demanding process and takes a toll on energy balance. Hence, energy homeostasis is a fundamental requirement in an organism's adaptive response to stress. The ability of an organism to tolerate and respond to stress is critical to its establishment and persistence in specific localities. This is particularly so in insects, which have successfully occupied most environmental niches and their continued success depends on responding effectively to and surviving a broad range of environmental stressors including temperature, desiccation, xenobiotic, osmotic and infection stress. In insects, the behavioral and physiological responses to diverse stressors are coordinated by the actions of various neurotransmitters and (neuro)hormones to facilitate stress induced changes ultimately leading to regulation of energy balance. Though the root cause of the mechanisms responsible for efficient energy homeostasis may remain contested, the central role of the brain in regulating energy balance remains undisputed. It could be argued that the emergence and evolution of the central nervous system is to promote the most effective means of dealing with energy homeostasis. Thus, the perception of stress leads to changes in the secretion profile of specific transmitters/hormones which essentially facilitate the modulation of physiology and behavior. Further, insulin-like peptides (ILPs) and adipokinetic hormones (AKHs) are neuropeptides that have similar roles as mammalian insulin and glucagon, respectively. The neurotransmitter dopamine (DA) has also been implicated in feeding and satiety responses bringing in possibilities of a complex neuro-regulatory network involved in energy homeostasis. These compounds - insulin, glucagon and increasingly also DA are critical components of metabolic pathways that regulate energy homeostasis in mammals. Dysfunctions in energy homeostasis mechanisms result in metabolic disorders such as obesity and diabetes in humans which represent a major public health challenge around the world. We explore the links between stress tolerance, metabolism, and energy balance using insects as model systems and demonstrate how in recent years, we have learned mostly from physiological responses in insects that many parallels exist between invertebrate and mammalian homeostasis. Thus, investigations on insects as simpler model organisms can provide useful information for elucidating the complexities of mammalian metabolism. An increased understanding of neural circuits underlying control of energy homeostasis is key for development of novel therapies in treatment of obesity and associated co-morbidities, including diabetes.

Keywords: adipokinetic hormone, insulin-like peptides, dopamine, energy homeostasis

1. INTRODUCTION

Energy homeostasis, or the homeostatic control of energy balance, is a biological process that involves the coordinated homeostatic regulation of energy inflow and energy expenditure. In other words it is a sensitive equilibrium kept between these two quantities with a tendency of a system to maintain *status quo* internally. Homeostasis is one of the most remarkable properties of complex systems that permit organisms to function effectively in a broad range of environmental conditions and allow survival against fluctuations such as availability of food and water, but also temperature, salinity, acidity etc. While the neural controls of cardiovascular and gastrointestinal functions have been intensively studied, the neural control of metabolism and particularly energy balance is less well understood and appreciated, probably owing to its complexity (Münzberg et al., 2016). Neural control of metabolism is accomplished by the coordinated actions on multiple levels including energy production, storage, mobilization, conversion and utilization. There are certain disorders that arise from dysfunctions in energy homeostasis mechanisms such as obesity, diabetes and associated disorders which represent a major public health challenge increasingly for the world. The physiological mechanisms that regulate energy balance are numerous. While the underlying cause of the mechanisms responsible for efficient energy storage are debatable, there is consensus that the brain plays a key role in regulating energy balance. It could be argued that the emergence and evolution of the central nervous system is to promote the most effective means of dealing with energy homeostasis. Thus, an increased understanding of neural circuits underlying control of energy homeostasis is key for development of novel therapies in treatment of obesity and associated co-morbidities, including diabetes.

In general, the ability of an organism to tolerate and respond to stress is critical to its establishment and persistence in specific localities, which is connected with the whole energy metabolism of an individual. This is particularly so in insects, which have successfully occupied most environmental niches and their continued success depends on responding effectively to and surviving a broad range of environmental stressors including temperature, desiccation, xenobiotic, osmotic and infection stress. In insects, the behavioral and physiological responses to diverse stressors are controlled by coordinated actions of neural and endocrine systems to facilitate stress induced changes (Johnson & White, 2009). Hence, the modulation of physiology and behavior occurs in response to changes in secretion profiles of specific transmitters/ hormones which is in turn related to the perception of stress.

2. NEURAL REGULATION OF ENERGY BALANCE AND HOMEOSTASIS

Neurotransmitters and neurohormones in insects serve as "master regulators" regulating almost all life processes including response to stress (Perić-Mataruga et al., 2006). The fruit fly *Drosophila melanogaster*, offers a genetically tractable model organism to understand pathways involved in energy homeostasis. *Drosophila* insulin-like peptides (DILPs) and adipokinetic hormones (AKHs) are neuropeptides that have similar roles as mammalian insulin and glucagon, respectively. Similarly, the neurotransmitter dopamine (DA) is known to be involved in the regulation of arousal, locomotor activity, mood and reward in mammals (Wise, 2002; Aarts et al., 2011) as well as in *Drosophila* (Pendleton et al., 2002; Andretic et al., 2005; Martin & Krantz, 2014). The insulin signaling pathway is highly conserved from *Drosophila* to mammals and performs essentially the same fundamental diverse physiological functions including the regulation of carbohydrate and lipid metabolism (Taguchi & White, 2008). ILPs are encoded by multigene families that are expressed in the brain and other tissues. Upon secretion, these peptides likely serve as hormones, neurotransmitters, and growth factors. In *D. melanogaster*, molecular genetic studies have revealed elements of a conserved insulin signaling pathway which appears to play a key role in metabolism, growth, reproduction, and aging (Wu & Brown, 2006). The insulin/insulin-like growth factor (IGF) signaling pathway is part of nutrient-sensing mechanisms that control growth, metabolism, reproduction, stress responses, and lifespan. So far, eight insulin-like peptides (DILP1-8) have been discovered in *Drosophila*. The insulin producing cells (IPCs) of the fly which are homologous to pancreatic beta cells are found in the brain (in the median neurosecretory cluster) (Rulifson et al., 2002), and produce at least three of the known DILP (DILP2, DILP3 and DILP5) (Ikeya et al., 2002). Ablation of these IPCs resulted in increased lipid and carbohydrate levels as well as increased resistance to starvation and oxidative stress (OS) (Broughton et al., 2005).

AKH is both synthesized and released from intrinsic endocrine cells of the *corpus cardiacum* (CC), a part of the ring gland in *Drosophila*. AKH has been implicated as being necessary and critical for maintenance of energy homeostasis (Bharucha et al., 2008; Braco et al., 2012). Moreover, dysregulation of glucose homeostasis is also observed when AKH-producing cells were ablated or when targeted mutagenesis of AKH hormone encoding gene was conducted (Kim & Rulifson, 2004; Lee & Park, 2004; Sajwan et al., 2015; Gáliková et al., 2015). These findings suggest that the insulin-glucagon system of mammals, and the DILP-AKH system of *Drosophila* may have analogous roles in regulating energy homeostasis. However, little is known about the genomic targets through which DILPs and AKH signaling act. A key question is whether these peptides regulate each other, so that only one type of peptide is dominantly produced under a certain physiological circumstance (related to energy homeostasis). Unpaired 2 (Upd2), a cytokine and a functional analogue of leptin and CCHamine-2, a nutrient responsive peptide hormone from fat body that remotely regulates physiological homeostasis by controlling insulin secretion has been reported in adult *Drosophila* (Rajan & Perrimon, 2012; Sano et al., 2015). Moreover, AKH expression is increased in larvae and adults of *Drosophila* lacking brain IPCs (Buch et al., 2008). However, the regulatory elements involving Upd2 as an energy sensor from fat body and as a proximate signal to AKH - the effector of lipid and carbohydrate mobilization in fat body tissues through DILPs - are as yet not defined.

Biogenic amines or catecholamines such as DA function as neurotransmitters and neurohormones and are reported to play key roles in orchestrating the response to stress in both vertebrates and invertebrates (Sabban, 2007; Hanna et al., 2015). Recently, it has also been found that DA has sexually dimorphic role in senescence in *D. melanogaster* (Bednářová et al., 2017). DA release from cells in several brain regions is stimulated in response to diverse stressors (D'Angio et al., 1988; Abercrombie et al., 1989). A temporally and sexually dimorphic recruitment of DA neurons into stress response circuitry has been reported in *Drosophila* (Argue et al., 2013a,b). However, the precise downstream signaling cascades activated in response to release of DA in its stress responsive role are as yet unclear. Does DA activate stress responsive pathways directly or indirectly through modulation of other neurohormones? A likely candidate for the latter is the AKH. While AKHs have originally been implicated in their roles in energy metabolism, presently it is accepted that AKHs play a pleiotropic role and have stress responsive functions (Kodrík, 2008; Krishnan & Kodrík, 2012; Bednářová et al., 2013, 2015; Bodláková et al., 2017). Given the roles of AKH as a neuroendocrine factor that regulates energetic status throughout insects, it is not surprising that AKH is also involved in stress response. The *"fight or flight"* response to stress requires the mobilization of energy sources to fuel the stress response and perhaps also activate signal cascades in stress response pathway as demonstrated recently (Bednářová et al., 2015; Gáliková et al., 2015).

It is evident that ILPs, AKH and DA play a critical role in energy homeostasis in insects, yet the connection among them is still unclear. There is a plethora of literature available on each of these three evolutionarily conserved compounds, however since everything is tightly integrated and connected together for a prompt response to energy imbalance caused by many different reasons, we expect that even signaling of these three compounds might be tightly connected. This review is targeted to uncover these links based on available literature in an effort to expand our knowledge on neuronal regulation of energy homeostasis. We will highlight how advances in understanding of the neurophysiology underlying metabolism including neural circuits using *D. melanogaster* as a model species may hold promise for development of therapies in the treatment of obesity, diabetes associated co-morbidities and neurodegenerative disorders.

3. INSULIN-LIKE PEPTIDES, ADIPOKINETIC HORMONES AND DOPAMINE IN INSECTS

3.1. Insulin-like Peptides, Signaling and Interaction with Other Transcription Factors and Modulators

Multiple aspects of growth, metabolic homeostasis, stress responses, fecundity and lifespan in *Drosophila* and other organisms are regulated by insulin and IGF signaling (IIS), a part of a nutrient – sensing pathway (Brogiolo et al., 2001; Broughton et al., 2005; Tatar et al., 2003; Grönke et al., 2010; Toivonen & Partridge, 2009; Fontana et al., 2010). The IIS pathway is largely conserved over evolution (Brogiolo et al., 2001; Teleman, 2010; Garofalo, 2002; Antonova et al., 2012), which makes *Drosophila* an excellent genetically tractable model system to investigate IIS mechanisms. As mentioned above eight DILP have been identified in *Drosophila* (Brogiolo et al., 2001; Grönke et al., 2010; Garelli et al., 2012; Colombani et al., 2012). Six of them have been studied in some detail with respect to their spatiotemporal expression patterns putative functions. DILP2, 3 and 5 are produced by a set of 14 median neurosecretory cells (IPCs) in the brain of larvae and adults (Brogiolo et al., 2001; Cao & Brown 2001; Rulifson et al., 2002). These DILPs are thought to be released into the open circulation from axon terminations in the *corpora cardiaca* and *corpora allata*, as well as on the surface of the anterior intestine and aorta (Cao & Brown 2001; Rulifson et al., 2002; Nässel et al., 2013; Park et al., 2014), and have been found sufficient for regulation of stress resistance, fecundity, metabolic homeostasis and lifespan (Brogiolo et al., 2001; Broughton et al., 2005; Rulifson et al., 2002; Ikeya et al., 2002; Padmanabha & Baker, 2014;

Owusu-Ansah & Perrimon 2014). DILP6, an IGF-like peptide, is produced mainly in the fat body and regulates growth during non-feeding stages (Slaidina et al., 2009; Okamoto et al., 2009). DILP7 is found in a set of about 20 neurons in the abdominal neuromeres of the ventral nerve cord of larvae and adults and plays roles in regulation of gut functions, tracheal growth and reproductive behavior (Miguel-Aliaga et al., 2008; Yang et al., 2008; Cognigni et al., 2011; Linneweber et al., 2014). DILP8 is released from the imaginal discs of larvae and can delay metamorphosis by inhibiting ecdysone biosynthesis, and thereby coordinates tissue growth with developmental timing (Garelli et al., 2012; Colombani et al., 2012). In adult flies DILP8 and its G-protein-coupled receptor Lgr3 play a role in reproduction (Meissner et al., 2016). Till date, not much is known about DILP1 and DILP4.

While in general it has been established that insulin regulates growth of essentially all tissues during the larval stage, however, its effect in adults is largely restricted to metabolic homeostasis, resistance to stress, fecundity and lifespan (Broughton et al., 2005; Grönke et al., 2010). Genetic ablation of the IPCs during early larval stages delays development and results in elevated sugar levels in the larval hemolymph (Rulifson et al., 2002); however, ablation during the adult stage results in reduced fecundity, increased storage of triglycerides and sugars, heightened resistance to starvation and OS, and prolonged lifespan (Broughton et al., 2005). Nevertheless, it is unclear whether the phenotypes associated with IPC ablation are due solely to the secreted ILPs or other peptides that IPCs can secrete as well. Regulation of insulin signaling in *Drosophila* is complex despite the fact that the core intracellular IIS cascade consists of single genes encoding the insulin-like receptor (InR), Akt (protein kinase B), phosphoinositide 3-kinase (PI3K) and forkhead transcription factor FoxO. Other than DILPs that regulate insulin signaling, there is a host of insulin-antagonizing peptides that have notable impacts on insulin signaling as well. Despite this, the insulin signal transduction pathway has well-characterized roles in the control of energy metabolism and tissue growth during animal development (for review, see Hafen, 2004). Activation of the InR leads to activation of PI3K, Akt, and finally TOR kinases through a relay of phosphorylation events. Cellular glucose and amino acid levels also independently regulate the TOR pathway, thereby integrating information about the nutritional status of the cell with that of the organism (Avruch et al., 2005). This signaling has two main output branches: one is transcriptional, via Akt-mediated phosphorylation, which inactivates FoxO-family transcription factors by promoting their cytoplasmic retention (Puig et al., 2003; Wolfrum et al., 2003). The second output controls cellular protein synthesis via TOR, which acts on 4E-BP and S6K, both important regulators of translation (Hay & Sonenberg, 2004). The control of fat metabolism in insects and mammals have been ascribed to the FoxO and TOR output branches of the insulin pathway (Wolfrum et al., 2004; Arquier et al., 2005; Reiling et al., 2005; Teleman et al., 2005b; Tettweiler et al., 2005). Finally, metabolic homeostasis also requires that organs coordinate their activities by means of the secretion of humoral factors or the propagation of nerve impulses between the organs. This phenomenon is a fairly well-established in mammalian systems, because the brain is known to process signals relating to the nutritional status of an organism and then elicit appropriate systemic responses. There are indications that *Drosophila* organs can also 'communicate' with each other, and recent studies in flies have revealed several inter-organ signaling modules, some of which are regulated by DILPs. For example, overexpression of FoxO in flight muscles was found to reduce both feeding behavior and insulin secretion from the IPCs. This in turn delays the accumulation of misfolded protein aggregates not only in muscles, but also non-autonomously in non-muscle tissue (Demontis & Perrimon, 2010). The fat body has also been shown to remotely control the secretion of DILPs from the IPCs through a mechanism dependent on the 'target of rapamycin' (TOR) (Colombani et al., 2003; Géminard et al., 2009). The existence of a humoral signal (or signals) released from the fat body that can impede the secretion of DILPs from the IPCs was proposed based on a series of elegant *ex vivo* cultures of larval brains and fat body tissue (Géminard et al., 2009). Eventually, Upd2, a specific ligand of the *Drosophila* JAK-STAT pathway, was found to be induced in the fat body during the fed state (Rajan & Perrimon, 2012). Interestingly, Upd2 induction in the fat body is also associated with the release of DILPs from the IPCs in the brain (Rajan & Perrimon, 2012). It has also been shown that DILP6 was upregulated in the fat body in response to fasting or FoxO overexpression and could also repress secretion of DILP2 from IPCs in the brain (Bai et al., 2012). Furthermore, overexpression of DILP6 in head or abdominal fat body caused many of the classic traits associated with downregulation of insulin signaling, such as the presence of increased whole-body triglycerides, stress resistance and lifespan of female flies (Bai et al., 2012). Thus, it will be of interest to investigate whether Upd2 and DILP6 act in concert or in parallel to regulate DILP secretion from IPCs. Moreover, involvement of AKH in these situations is highly possible as well, since AKH plays a critical role in energy metabolism and also stress resistance (Bednářová et al., 2013, 2015). More about the AKH signaling is discussed in the subsequent section (3.2.).

The role of FoxO factors in mediating nutritional programming of lifespan is evolutionarily conserved between worms and flies, making it likely that they play an equivalent role in nutritional programming in mammals. Recently, an interesting study was published by Dobson et al. (2017), where they conducted an elegant set of experiments which implicated that FoxO factors is the missing mechanistic link between early-life nutrition and longevity. The strong evolutionary conservation of FoxO function makes it highly likely that FoxO factors play a role in some aspect of nutritional programming in mammals. The role of *Drosophila* FoxO in mediating the long-term effects of a sugar-rich diet in *Drosophila* is surprisingly specific. FoxO is not required for the lifespan benefits of a chronic reduction in protein intake, even though its activity can modulate the response (Giannakou et al., 2008). Similarly, the survival of *foxo*-null flies is reduced by chronic feeding with a sugar-rich diet to the same extent as the wild-type's (Al Saud et al., 2015). These differences in the role of FoxO in response to chronic or acute dietary regimes, or different dietary components, may arise from the complex interactions between nutrition and insulin/IGF-like signaling: each DILP is expressed in a unique tissue pattern, acts in an endocrine and/or paracrine manner, and responds distinctly to the relative amounts of protein and carbohydrate present in the diet (Post & Tatar, 2016; Dobson et al., 2017). This, in turn, may specify the tissues in which FoxO is inhibited by specific diets and the nature of FoxO targets affected. FoxO is inhibited by the signaling cascade initiated by DILPs (Teleman, 2009). Dobson et al. (2017) found that one of these, *DILP6* was induced after one week of feeding on a sugar rich diet. Such an increase in insulin/IGF signaling is expected to result in phosphorylation and inhibition of FoxO (Brunet et al., 1999; Alic et al., 2011). Indeed, they found that FoxO phosphorylation was increased on a sugar rich diet. Hence, sugar-rich diet induces *DILP6* and inhibits FoxO to repress FoxO target genes, including epigenetic modifiers. Based on studies so far, it is obvious that the neuroendocrine architecture and IIS events in *Drosophila* are remarkably complex. Moreover, it is very essential to study the developmental context of hormone interactions since these kind of studies may reveal fundamental features of maintaining energy homeostasis which have important consequences for understanding not only metabolic disorders but also neurodegenerative diseases which are spread across our population.

3.2. Adipokinetic Hormone, Signaling and Interaction with Other Transcription Factors and Modulators

AKH is an insect neuropeptide produced by the *corpora cardiaca*, pair neurohemal organs, sometimes fused together, that are situated near the insect brain. AKH mobilizes carbohydrates and lipids from the insect fat body which is an organ comparable to the mammalian liver and adipose tissue, during high physical activities, such as insect flight and locomotion (Gäde et al., 1997; Kim & Rulifson, 2004). Thus, although not structurally related, AKH has the same functions in insects as glucagon and adrenalin have in mammals (Bednářová et al., 2013). AKH was one of the first neuropeptides to be purified and sequenced from insects, particularly from the locust *Locusta migratoria* (Stone et al., 1976). Since then, AKHs have been characterized in a large number of insect species and turned out to have rather variable structures. Generally, the following hallmarks for AKH structures can be deduced: (i) a length of 8, 9, or 10 amino acid residues; (ii) a pQ group in position 1; (iii) an aliphatic or aromatic amino acid residue in position 2; (iv) aromatic amino acid residues in positions 4; (v) a W residue in position 8; and (vi) either a Wamide, WGamide, or WGXamide C terminus (Gäde et al., 1997; Li et al., 2016). It has been suggested by Li et al. (2016) to call these AKH peptides "true AKHs", because during genomic and EST database mining other AKHs that were 10 amino-acid residues long and that had a WXGamide or WXPamide C terminus were discovered. The authors termed those peptides as "AKH-like". A third group of AKH-resembling peptides are the "proto-AKHs". They are longer than 10 amino acid residues, resemble AKHs, but have only 2–4 of the above-mentioned AKH hallmarks (Li et al., 2016). In 1998, a G protein-coupled receptor (GPCR) from *D. melanogaster* was characterized being structurally closely related to the mammalian gonadotropin releasing hormone (GnRH) receptor (Hauser et al., 1998). Four years later a ligand for this receptor from *Drosophila* larvae was determined; this was surprisingly not a GnRH-like peptide, but *Drosophila* AKH (Staubli et al., 2002). This discovery was the first finding indicating that an evolutionary link exists between insect AKH and vertebrate GnRH signaling. There are two other insect receptors that are structurally closely related to the AKH receptors: corazonin and the AKH/corazonin-related peptide (ACP) receptors (Belmont et al., 2006; Hansen et al., 2010). Also the ligands, corazonin and ACP, share several identical and conserved amino acid residues with AKH, suggesting receptor-ligand co-evolution of these three signaling systems (Belmont et al., 2006; Hansen et al., 2010). These findings also implicate that all three insect receptors are evolutionarily closely related to the vertebrate GnRH receptors. Interestingly, the insect AKH receptors are specific for AKH only, and are not activated by ACP or corazonin. Similarly, the ACP receptors are specific for ACP, and the corazonin receptors for corazonin, showing that AKH, ACP, and corazonin are three independent signaling systems (Shi et al., 2011). Discovery of functional AKH receptors in mollusks in the work of Li and co-workers (2016) is especially significant, because it traces the emergence of AKH signaling back to about 550 million years ago and brings us closer to a more complete understanding of the evolutionary origins of the GnRH receptor superfamily.

Like some other neuropeptides, AKHs are multifunctional. Other known physiological effects observed for those peptides in insects include cardioacceleration, increasing of muscle tonus and general locomotion, stimulation of immune response and digestive processes, inhibition of egg maturation and regulation of starvation-induced foraging behavior (for details see review Kodrík, 2008). AKHs also induce transcription of the cytochrome *P450* gene, expression of a gene encoding fatty acid binding protein and control a number of biochemical actions via stimulation/ inhibition of activity of responsible enzymes. In addition, AKH peptides have excitatory effects on motor neurons and might be involved into the neuronal signaling (Kodrík et al., 2015a); furthermore AKHs enhance amplitudes of the electroretinogram in the crayfish (Lee & Park 2004).

Recent evidence indicates that AKH may exert its role in response to oxidative stress (OS) (Kodrík et al., 2007) through activation of FoxO (Bednářová et al., 2015) which has been implicated in stress response, aging etc. The mechanism by which FoxO confers OS resistance is not yet known. Jünger et al. (2003) identified several genes encoding cytochrome P450 enzymes (Cyp4e2) as FoxO target gene candidates. Glauser & Schlegel (2007) proposed in their work that genes like *manganase superoxide dismutase* (*MnSOD*) and *catalase* (*CAT*) might be employed by FoxO, too, and therefore they partially mediate the protective effect of FoxO. This suggests that the anti-OS activities of FoxO are mainly attributable to their ability to induce the expression of anti-oxidant genes.

The precise pathway by which FoxO signaling may be activated, and its relationship to AKH, remains hypothetical at this point in time. It is also important to highlight that there might be other players and factors involved, which adds an additional layer of complexity to the whole process of AKH signaling during a situation of OS. Little is known about the genomic targets through which AKH signaling acts. It is plausible that in the fruit flies ILP signaling and AKH signaling are closely linked (Buch et al., 2008), and such signaling by AKH might involve FoxO as a mediator, particularly in its role in the anti-OS response. The paracrine and endocrine effects of AKH in response to OS are largely unexplored and might involve multiple targets and genes; the whole pathway might be more complex than is now assumed.

Further studies would be necessary to pinpoint the precise mechanism by which FoxO and AKH signaling might interact in maintenance of homeostasis by responding to OS.

3.3. Dopamine Signaling and Interaction with Other Transcription Factors and Modulators

Dopamine (DA) is a catecholamine, highly conserved throughout evolution (Yamamoto et al., 2014). In mammals, DA plays key roles in motor coordination as well as motivation, reward, addiction, learning, and memory. Dysregulation of DA signaling has been implicated in a variety of human disorders (Yamamoto et al., 2011). Most notably, loss of dopaminergic neurons is the principal defect in Parkinson's disease. The role of DA dysfunction as a consequence of OS, is involved in health and disease. In insects DA has a role in anti-immune defense system, in molting, metamorphosis and other processes Neckameyer (1996).

Components of DA biosynthesis are highly conserved across a divergent range of animal phyla and have been well described in mammalian and *Drosophila* systems (Barron et al., 2010). DA synthesis requires closely regulated cooperation of two enzymatic pathways, and is highly sensitive to external cues. In *D. melanogaster*, tyrosine hydroxylase (TH), encoded by the gene pale, converts tyrosine to DA during catecholamine synthesis (Neckameyer & White, 1993). TH catalytic activity requires and is regulated by the cofactor, tetrahydrobiopterin (BH4). The enzyme GTP cyclohydrolase I (GTPCH) is the initiating and limiting component of BH4 biosynthesis and therefore also in DA production (Hsouna et al., 2007). Once catecholamines such as DA are produced, they can be transported by vesicular monoamine transporters (VMAT) from the cytoplasm into synaptic vesicles (Greer et al., 2005).

In mammal, DA mediated triggering of transcription factors such as c-fos, and neuropeptide genes, such as prodynorphin in the rat striatum have been demonstrated (Hyman et al., 1995). It was shown that phosphorylation of transcription factor CREB (cAMP response element-binding protein) is a critical early event coupling DA stimulation to gene regulation. CREB interacts with functional regulatory elements in both the c-fos and prodynorphin genes, and is phosphorylated in response to DA in a D1 dopamine receptor-dependent manner (Hyman et al., 1995). Such studies are still in a nascent state in *Drosophila* though DA's interaction with other modulators such as octopamine has been demonstrated and its reciprocal links with FoxO (Gruntenko et al., 2016).

4. INSULIN-LIKE PEPTIDES, AKH AND DOPAMINE IN FEEDING BEHAVIOR

Feeding and energy metabolism is a basic and vital life process essential for individual and consequently species survival. It could be argued that the emergence and evolution of nervous system is to promote the most effective means of dealing with feeding and metabolism in support of survival. Accumulating experimental evidence is in agreement with this basic assertion. Thus, it is not unreasonable to claim that even higher brain regions, such as the archi- and neocortex, emerged under environmental pressures to support behaviors that more effectively deal with available energy resources. The pursuit to understand the role that the brain plays in the control of body energy balance has continued for more than a century (Gao & Horvath, 2008).

The function of IIS in growth control is remarkably conserved in insects, and in particular in *Drosophila*. A major role for IIS in insects is to couple growth with the animal's energy status. Indeed, total nutrient deprivation downregulates *DILP3* and *DILP5* transcription in the IPCs, although *DILP2* expression remains unchanged (Ikeya et al., 2002). Recent results indicate that variations in nutritional information are relayed by a nutrient sensor operating in the fat body. In particular, it has been shown that amino acid restriction triggers fat body-specific inhibition of the TOR complex1 (TORC1) (Colombani et al., 2003), a major cell-based nutrient-sensing pathway (Dann & Thomas, 2006; Wullschleger et al., 2006; Guertin &

Sabatini, 2007). Inhibition of TORC1 in the fat body systemically reduces larval growth in part by blocking DILP secretion from the brain IPCs (Géminard et al., 2009). Therefore, in line with the decreased levels of circulating IGF-I in vertebrates, starvation affects *Drosophila* growth by severely reducing brain-specific DILP function. Moreover, some DILP7-producing neurons innervate the adult hindgut and regulate feeding behavior in response to nutrient availability (Miguel-Aliaga et al., 2008; Cognigni et al., 2011; Owusu-Ansah & Perrimon, 2014). It has been shown that, in addition to their established role in DILP secretion, IPCs also secrete drososulfakinins, which act as a satiety signal by regulating both food choice and intake (Söderberg et al., 2012). These observations underscore the complexity of appetite regulation through peptidergic signaling and emphasize the need to study this phenomenon in a combinatorial context (Owusu-Ansah & Perrimon, 2014).

Starvation and feeding are intimately related. The majority of studies that examined the regulation of starvation stress has involved the insulin receptor signaling (IRS) pathway, which is well conserved between mammals and *Drosophila* (Britton et al., 2002). During conditions of low nutrient availability (e.g., amino acid starvation) the IRS signaling pathway is muted. With less insulin, more trehalose is present in the hemolymph, and this is coupled with an increase in lifespan (Broughton et al., 2008). The transcription factor FoxO, a downstream effector that is negatively regulated by insulin receptor activity, is more active when IRS decreases. Moreover, FoxO is important to survival during amino acid starvation (Kramer et al., 2008). *Drosophila* exposed to amino acid starvation media showed an increase in *foxo* expression, while the loss of FoxO activity resulted in decreased survivorship when flies were only fed sucrose without protein or amino acids. The neuropeptide regulation of feeding is associated with this mechanism, because the cell surface of specific *Drosophila* neurons contains both the NPF receptor and the insulin receptor (Wu et al., 2006). When IRS is lowered in these neurons, larvae will overeat (including foods they would normally avoid). However, when there was an increase in IRS in these neurons, the larvae eat far less than expected. This suggests that the IRS negatively regulates the action of the NPF receptor, and thus NPF signaling in *Drosophila*.

As mentioned also above, AKHs also control locomotion (Socha et al., 1999; Kodrík et al., 2000) and feeding (Kodrík et al., 2012), and additionally both these responses together: locomotor behavior in response to starvation (Isabel et al., 2005; Lee & Park, 2004). After a period of food deprivation wild-type flies become hyperactive. This increased locomotor activity may reflect an attempt to find food after decreasing energy reserves, and thus an essential behavioral constituent since food is not constantly available in a natural environment. Genetically ablating the AKH cells yields flies where this starvation-induced hyperactivity is absent. The lack of hyperactivity in the AKH-ablated flies is suggested to lead to the conservation of energy and thus explain the increased survival at starvation that these flies display. Hence, during starvation AKH is suggested to regulate both metabolic (sugar and lipid homeostasis) and behavioral (starvation-induced hyperactivity) functions and thus increase the fly's chances of survival when food is scarce (Isabel et al., 2005). It has been suggested that the AKH-mediated hyperactivity is not a direct physiological effect of sugar levels (that are lower in AKH-ablated flies). Instead AKH is proposed to directly modify locomotor activity, since circulating trehalose levels in the AKH-ablated flies still are high enough to allow normal locomotion (Isabel et al., 2005; Lee and Park, 2004). Furthermore, AKH over expression elevates sugar levels but do not alter locomotor activity.

Gáliková et al. (2016) conducted extensive studies on the physiological cause of the AKH deficiency-triggered obesity, they hypothesized that the obese phenotype might result from excessive feeding. Therefore, they monitored food intake of the *Akh^A* (loss-of-AKH-function) and *AkhR^1* (loss-of-AKH-receptor-function) mutants during the first week of adulthood but surprisingly, they found out that *Akh^A* and *AkhR^1* mutations actually decrease food intake. Consistently, increase in the AKH signaling by over-expression of *Akh* caused hypophagia. Their results suggests that AKH signaling affects feeding independently of its anti-obesity roles in the fat body. Their data showed that despite being an anti-obesity hormone, *Drosophila* AKH is an orexigenic peptide, and the AKH deficiency results in obesity without hyperphagia. Altogether, their work shows that *Drosophila* AKH signaling has multiple metabolic functions and the deficiency for AKH affects energy homeostasis in several ways, including regulation of feeding, metabolism, and expression of metabolic regulators from the neuropeptide hormone family, including the fly ILPs.

The mammalian midbrain DA system is known to be involved in the regulation of arousal, locomotor activity, mood, and reward. DA deficiency in mice, generated by selective inactivation of tyrosine hydroxylase, markedly suppressed food intake (Szczypka et al., 1999). These mice fail to eat in response to acute glucose deprivation, suggesting that DA signaling is absolutely required for promoting feeding and acts downstream of the melanocortin system (Hnasko et al., 2004). Moreover, a neural hormone regulator, the DA transporter (DAT), works to clear DA from the synapses. This action may manipulate the post-feeding reward circuit in that lowered DA levels depress feeding, and excess DA levels encourage feeding (Slade & Staveley, 2016). The DA neurotransmitter functions in reward-motivated behaviors; thus, changes to extracellular DA levels can result in a number of diseases (Palmiter, 2007; Yamamoto & Seto, 2014). Low levels of DA are associated with attention deficit hyperactivity disorder, depression, and under-eating (Sotak et al., 2005). Studies in rats showed that upon feeding or drinking, there was a rapid firing of DA in the brain. However, animals with lowered or no DA activity were hypoactive, apparently apathetic, and prone to death from starvation or dehydration (Schultz, 2006). Conversely, hyper-dopaminergic mice overfed and eventually became obese (Cagniard et al., 2006). Therefore, manipulation of the transporter that regulates the strength and duration of DA signaling could lead to similar outcomes. The *Drosophila DAT* gene was re-isolated in a screen for genes that alter sleep (Kume et al., 2005). A *DAT* mutant, named fumin (*fmn*) (Japanese for sleepless), is active for nearly 24 hours in a day. *Drosophila DAT* expression patterns were concentrated in known dopaminergic neuron locations within larvae and the adult head. Overall, it is evident that DA activity could be an effective regulator of feeding. When DAT, a member of the post-feeding reward system, is either overexpressed or reduced via mutation, *Drosophila* has increased sensitivity to amino acid starvation. Taken together, these results indicate that subtle variation in the expression of key components of these systems impacts survivorship during adverse nutrient conditions.

5. ROLE OF INSULIN-LIKE PEPTIDES, AKH AND DOPAMINE IN RESPONSE TO HOMEOSTATIC CHALLENGES

All living organisms respond to stressful changes of the environment in strikingly various ways. However, with all the diversity of responses to stress at both the cell level and the level of the organism, the major task is to overcome the effects of the influencing factor and increase the organism resistance. Neurohormones are the master regulators of all life processes in insects and employ a strategy of triggering stress-protective events. A stressor signal received by an insect's receptors is transmitted via sensory nerves to the brain, whose neurons (having processed the information and assessed the stimulation level as extreme) transmit a message along cardiac nerves calling for urgent release of neurohormones synthesized in neurosecretory cells and stored in the neurohemal organs. The first stress reaction, depending on speed of the metabolic response, is linked with the secretion of biogenic amines (Davenport & Evans, 1984). Under their influence, within a few minutes the reserve energy substrates are mobilized. In the subsequent phase of the stress responsive process, a more complex set of physiological reactions takes place. Its first stage is realized by neurohormones primarily by interaction of adipokinetic neurohormones ILPs in concert with biogenic amines.

5.1. Insulin-like Peptides in Response to Homeostatic Challenge

Insulin/IFG signaling pathway controls stress tolerance and metabolic homeostasis in higher organisms, influencing lifespan (Tatar & Yin, 2001; Russell & Kahn, 2007; Taguchi & White, 2008), but the mechanism(s) by which IIS activity is modulated in response to stress remain to be established. Recent work in flies, worms, and mice suggest that stress signaling pathways play an important role in this regulation, increasing lifespan, and stress tolerance by repressing IIS activity (Oh et al., 2005; Wang et al., 2005; Schumacher et al., 2008). Interestingly, a similar antagonism between stress signaling and IIS also seems to be central to the etiology of type II diabetes, suggesting that repression of IIS activity is an important acute response to stress, but has deleterious effects on metabolic homeostasis under chronic conditions (Hotamisligil, 2006). In particular, the stress-responsive Jun-N-terminal Kinase (JNK) pathway has been shown to regulate IIS activity at multiple levels, influencing lifespan and stress tolerance in lower organisms and promoting insulin resistance in mouse models for diabetes (Hirosumi et al., 2002; Oh et al., 2005; Wang et al., 2005; Karpac & Jasper, 2009). JNK can repress IIS signal transduction by phosphorylating the insulin receptor substrate, as well as by activating the IIS-regulated transcription factor FoxO, but can also interfere with ILP expression in IPCs (Hirosumi et al., 2002; Essers et al., 2004; Oh et al., 2005; Wang et al., 2005). It has been found out that ablation of IPCs results in flies with diabetic phenotypes, but extended lifespan and increased stress tolerance (Rulifson et al., 2002; Broughton et al., 2005), and repressing ILP expression in IPCs by over-expression of either the JNK Kinase Hemipterous (Hep), or a dominant-negative version of p53 results in increased lifespan (Wang et al., 2005; Bauer et al., 2007). While these studies confirm that forced repression of ILP expression is sufficient to impair IIS activity and increase stress tolerance and longevity, it remains unclear whether this repression is part of an acute adaptive response to environmental stress. Nevertheless, Karpac & Jasper (2009), showed that IPC-specific JNK activity is required for ILP repression in response to OS in flies, mediating stress-induced growth repression during development and promoting adult stress tolerance. They proved that IPC-specific JNK signaling is central to systemic adaptive responses to acute environmental challenges.

In the fruitfly *Drosophila* genetic ablation of cells in the brain producing ILPs, or mutations in the ILP receptor (dInR) and other insulin signaling components, lead to an increase in stress tolerance and extension of life span at the expense of fertility and body size (Baker & Thummel, 2007; Giannakou & Partridge, 2007; Teleman, 2010). Also carbohydrate and lipid homeostasis is affected by these manipulations (Rulifson et al., 2002; Baker & Thummel, 2007). Although much has been learned about insulin signaling downstream of the insulin receptor, it is not clear how the production and release of DILPs is regulated in adult *Drosophila* in response to nutritional or stress signals (Geminard et al., 2006). Nutritional sensing appears to take place in adipose tissue, the fat body (Colombani et al., 2003) and recently it was shown that there is a humoral link between the fat body and insulin-producing cells (IPCs) in the brain (Geminard et al., 2009). Thus, availability of nutrients sensed by the fat body is an important factor in regulation of DILP release. In addition recent evidence suggest that the IPCs can sense glucose levels autonomously (Kreneisz et al., 2010). It is likely that hormonal or neural signals also regulate production and release of DILPs by IPCs of the adult insect, as has been shown to be the case in pancreatic beta-cells in mammals (Drucker et al., 1987; Sonoda et al, 2008).

However, such hormones have not yet been identified in the fly, although recently neurons expressing, short neuropeptide F, GABA (gamma-aminobutyric acid) or serotonin were suggested as regulators of DILP production in IPCs of the brain (Lee et al., 2008; Enell et al., 2010). The roles of DILPs in stress resistance and regulation of life span are well established in *Drosophila* (Giannakou & Partridge, 2007), but hormonal mechanisms for regulation of production and release of DILPs in IPCs of adult flies have not been reported. However, Söderberg et al. (2011) were able to demonstrate that of DTKs act on IPCs in the renal tubules which is a first identification of a hormonal factor regulating DILP release in adult insects. Also OS resistance is linked to insulin signaling in *Drosophila* (Giannakou & Partridge, 2007; Kabil et al., 2007). Superoxide dismutases (SOD) are key enzymes protecting proteins from reactive oxygen species and are thought to be regulated by insulin signaling: SOD activity is elevated in chico (dInR substrate) mutants of *Drosophila* (Kabil et al., 2007). Also in yeast insulin-signaling mutations affect lifespan via SOD (Fabrizio et al., 2001). Söderberg et al. (2011) also found that knockdown of Sod2 (encoding MnSOD), but not Sod1, in renal tubules decreased lifespan at desiccation and OS in *Drosophila*. Thus, it is possible that DILP signaling in tubules target mitochondrial SOD2 and affects resistance to OS. Interestingly, diminishing OS resistance via Sod2 locally in the principal cells of *Drosophila* renal tubules is sufficient to shorten the lifespan of the fly during stress (Söderberg et al., 2011).

5.2. AKH Regulation of Response to Homeostatic Challenge

In mammals, the stress response pathways are controlled from the hypothalamic–pituitary brain center with the help of a suite of corresponding hormones. In insects, the anti-OS reactions seem to be regulated predominantly by AKHs (Kodrík et al., 2015b). Indeed, recently published work using the *Drosophila* model system presented evidence that AKH may primarily employ the FoxO to exert its effect in protection of the organism against OS (Bednářová et al., 2015). In *D. melanogaster dFoxO* proteins are expressed predominantly in fat body and play an important mediatory role in the insulin signaling pathway, which adjusts growth and metabolism to nutrient availability. The insulin signaling pathway and AKH-stimulated cAMP signaling pathway also seem to be linked, or they use similar mechanisms to orchestrate the organism's response to both nutritional conditions and stress. Findings from the work of Bednářová et al. (2015) are consistent with the idea that there may be a link between these two signaling pathways or they could act in concert when facing a stress situation.

5.3. Dopamine Regulated Response to Homeostatic Challenge

Control of stress response includes both neural and endocrine levels. The biogenic amine DA is a component that links both of them. So, the catecholamine signaling pathway is highly important component of the stress response. In *Drosophila* DA levels are significantly elevated under heat, nutrition, mechanical stress and OS (Hanna et al., 2015). Cell stress signaling pathways, including oxidative stress and starvation also stimulate

FoxO (Jünger et al., 2003; Hwangbo et al., 2004). Under normal conditions, FoxO is inactive, inhibited by IIS; in the absence of IIS, in particular during nutrient deprivation, FoxO translocates to the nucleus where it activates gene expression (Jünger et al., 2003; Puig et al., 2003). The environmental stressors are also known to cause changes in the expression of hundreds of genes (Lopez-Maury et al., 2008). An alternative mechanism to regulate the activity of FoxO appears to occur through the juvenile hormone (JH) (Mirth et al., 2014). FoxO activity is significantly higher in *D. melanogaster* larvae with genetically ablated *corpora allata*, the organ that produces JH (Mirth et al., 2014). Overexpression of FoxO increases OS tolerance (Hwangbo et al., 2004) while FoxO -null mutants are more sensitive to OS (Jünger et al., 2003) and deficient in viral defense (Spellberg & Marr, 2015). Grutenko et al. (2016) using *Drosophila* mutants where expression of FoxO was declined, demonstrated dramatic changes in the metabolism of DA and octopamine and so the overall stress response. Their findings suggest that FoxO is a possible trigger for endocrinological stress reactions. Neckameyer (1996) showed that increased levels of DA were accompanied by a decrease in the activity of the enzyme tyrosine hydroxylase (TH), that catalyzes the first and rate limiting step in DA synthesis, when exposed to stress. Grutenko et al. (2016) also found out that shortage of FoxO in one-day-old females caused a decline in both the synthesis and degradation of DA. Under normal conditions, the activity of ALP (alkaline phosphatase enzyme), TH and DA-dependent arylalkylamine N-acetyltransferase (DAT) in FoxO deficit female flies was decreased compared with controls. In addition, the stress reactivity of enzymes in the DA synthesis pathway was reduced. Their data also suggest that DA levels in young FoxO-deficit females are elevated which is consistent with their previous study showing that DA downregulates the activity of its synthesis enzymes (Bogomolova et al., 2010). Low levels of DAT activity may cause an increase in DA levels, which in turn could decrease ALP and TH activity. The decreased DAT activity in FoxO deficit females may be due to decreased levels of JH. Previous studies have shown that JH metabolism is disrupted in FoxO deficit females (Rauschenbach et al., 2015) and that JH regulates DA content via DAT in young *Drosophila* females (Rauschenbach et al., 2014). Overall, it seems that stress triggers the response of FoxO, which triggers an increase in JH titer, in turn modifying the metabolism of biogenic amines. It is expected that FoxO confers oxidative-stress resistance via the transcriptional upregulation of genes encoding anti-oxidative enzymes.

In our recent work (Hanna et al., 2015) we monitored the impact of mutations in four essential genes involved in dopamine (DA) synthesis and transport on longevity, motor behavior, and resistance to OS in *D. melanogaster*. We hypothesize that DA could directly influence GSTO1 transcription and thus play a significant role in the regulation of response to OS. Interestingly, DA is also a self-oxidizing catecholamine known to generate reactive oxygen species including hydrogen peroxide, making catecholaminergic neurons extremely susceptible to higher OS and more free radical damage than other types of neurons (Hald & Lotharius, 2005). Catecholamines up (Catsup), works as a negative regulator of DA production that acts on TH and GTPCH, both of which are rate-limiting enzymes (Stathakis et al., 1999). Moreover, loss-of-function mutations in Catsup hyperactivate TH by a post-translational mechanism that also corresponds to increased catecholamine pool levels. Paradoxically, Catsup mutants are resistant to OS induced by paraquat (Chaudhuri et al., 2007) and have also been reported to cause dominant hyperactivation of both TH as well as GTPCH (Wang et al., 2011). The latter study also established that VMAT was hyperactivated by Catsup, and the excess DA is both transported into synaptic vesicles and released into the synapse at higher rates in Catsup mutants. However, reasons behind the resistance of Catsup mutants to OS remains unclear. DA has been shown to be a marker of neuronal senescence in *Drosophila*, since its levels decrease with increasing age, accompanied by deficits in dopaminergic modulated behaviors in aging flies (Neckameyer et al., 2000). In our recent work Hanna et al. (2015) we observed a differential response to OS in the expression of Cu/Zn SOD, MnSOD, and GSTO3 in DA mutants. Over-expression of Cu/Zn SOD has been demonstrated to protect dopaminergic neurons in *Drosophila* (Botella et al., 2008), however, in the work of Hanna et al. (2015), any significant up-regulation of Cu/Zn SOD associated with increased tolerance to OS was not observed. While we quantified the gene expression patterns of five major anti-oxidant enzymes, we were able to target protein quantitation of only two anti-oxidative enzymes viz. MnSOD and GSTO1 since reliable antibodies were available only for them. Among the two, only glutathione S-transferase Omega 1 (GSTO1) gene expression and its protein levels indicated that elevated DA pools could be triggering an up-regulation in the expression of this gene along with enhanced activity.

Moreover, DA signaling, strongly influenced by DAT activity, is linked to IRS, because the insulin receptor is expressed in the dopaminergic neurons of the midbrain of *Drosophila* (Palmiter, 2007; Mebel et al., 2012). Inhibition of the receptor reduces IRS and *DAT* expression; hence, DA clearance and the administration of insulin directly to the rat brain (via intracerebroventricular administration) lead to increases in *DAT* mRNA and activity that clear the synapses and decrease DA levels (Figlewicz et al., 1994). Rats fed a high-fat diet have decreased levels of Akt1 activity in the brain, and they require a longer period to clear the synapses of DA (Speed et al., 2011). Upon addition of the insulin receptor substrate, Akt1 levels are restored, and expression of DAT on the cell surfaces in the striatum is also reestablished. Other hormones that homeostatically control feeding behavior have also been shown to interact with receptors on neurons that secrete DA. Leptin, an anorexigenic hormone, inhibits DA activity, while ghrelin (an orexin) stimulates DA activity to influence the reward potential of feeding (Palmiter, 2007). Since lowered IRS and increased FoxO activity are pertinent to the maximized survival of *Drosophila* undergoing amino acid starvation (Kramer et al., 2008), it would be expected that reduced DAT would result in the same phenotype, while overexpression of *dat* would impair survival. However, we found that both upregulation and reduced activity of DAT decreased survivorship when flies were starved of amino acids.

It is clear that manipulation of components associated with the homeostatic control of stress situations affect survival during adverse nutrient and overall ambient conditions. While it is expected that overexpression some components should yield opposite results compared to lowering or loss of function experiments, this is not always observed. Many results indicated that it is important to maintain a sensitive balance in order to appropriately regulate the complex behavior while facing stress situations, so that survivorship during adverse nutrient and ambient conditions can be maximized.

6. REGULATION OF ENERGY HOMEOSTASIS BY INSULIN-LIKE PEPTIDES, AKH AND DOPAMINE

The mechanisms that control energy homeostasis and tissue growth during development are closely linked through several signal transduction pathways. Changes in the level of insulin and AKH reflect the nutritional status of the organism to control circulating sugar levels and fat metabolism. Systemic defects in insulin responsiveness can lead to elevated circulating glucose levels and fat accumulation. In mammals, the peptide hormones insulin and glucagon are critical for regulation of blood-glucose levels and energy availability (Unger & Cherrington, 2012). *Drosophila* possess functional orthologs of insulin and glucagon that appear to have conserved roles in the regulation of metabolic function (Edgar, 2006). The glucagon ortholog AKH is expressed in the CC (Kim & Rulifson, 2004; Lee & Park, 2004). The CC receives input from insulin IPCs and secretes AKH into the hemolymph (Rulifson et al., 2002; Kim & Rulifson, 2004). Ablation of the CC results in hypoglycemia, highlighting the importance of these cells in glucose sensing and overall metabolic regulation (Kim & Rulifson, 2004). Manipulations that impair AKH signaling promote glycogen and triglyceride storage, confirming a role for this pathway in controlling carbohydrate and fat metabolism (Kim & Rulifson, 2004; Lee & Park, 2004; Isabel et al., 2005). AKH function is also implicated in a number of behaviors associated with hunger-induced motivation, including odor-conditioned feeding approach, feeding, and locomotor behavior (Lee & Park, 2004; Burt et al., 2014). Ablation of AKH-producing cells reduces the hyperlocomotor and feeding responses to starvation and increases starvation resistance (Lee & Park, 2004; Bharucha et al., 2008). Therefore, AKH signaling potently regulates behavior in response to starvation, but it is unclear whether these changes are due to altered energy stores or the acute effects of AKH function.

In *Drosophila* many behavioral processes are controlled by ILP (Rulifson et al., 2002; DiAngelo & Birnbaum, 2009). For example in *Drosophila* larvae, both *ilp3* and *ilp5* are transcriptionally downregulated in response to starvation, suggesting a role in nutritional state-dependent regulation of behavior and metabolism (Ikeya et al., 2002). Generally, ILPs bind to a single insulin-like receptor (dInR), which is proposed to express ubiquitously (Fernandez et al., 1995). Unlike all other *ilps*, *ilp6* is predominantly expressed in the liver/adipose tissue-like organ, the fat body, raising the possibility that insulin signaling in the fat body is auto-regulated (Okamoto et al., 2009). Activating insulin signaling specifically in the fat body promotes fat storage similar to mammals (DiAngelo & Birnbaum, 2009). Therefore, ILPs and AKH have diverse functions in regulating metabolism and behavior.

The role of DA in energy metabolism and behavior is much less clear, however, in the light of its role in feeding behavior, it can be assumed that DA may have crucial function in energy homeostasis (Slade & Staveley, 2016). The act of feeding by any organism must be modified based on the environment and available nutrition in order to maintain an appropriate energy balance. A disruption in this balance may lead to metabolic diseases, including obesity and eating disorders such as anorexia (Fairburn & Harrison, 2003). A myriad of genes helps maintain this balance by prompting foraging and feeding, or by encouraging the cessation of feeding. Expression of these genes is often triggered by internal mechanisms that monitor the levels of peripheral energy stores. When there is sufficient energy stored, anorexic genes can signal satiety to cause the organism to stop feeding. When internal energy stores are lowered, the orexic genes can signal to the organism that feeding is necessary to restore energy. Typically this homeostatic process, which in mammals measures energy stores and relays signals between the hypothalamus and the periphery (Hoebel, 1971), works efficiently. However, in an environment where nutrients are readily available, an additional post-satiation reward system can regulate feeding patterns. Although the homeostatic response works well when animals are required to forage, the post-satiation reward can override the homeostatic signals when there is an excess of food (Palmiter, 2007). Thus, it has been convincingly demonstrated in *Drosophila* that manipulating the DA system has an impact on feeding behavior and its sensitivity to amino acid starvation (Slade & Staveley, 2016).

7. CONCLUSION AND FUTURE PERSPECTIVES: DYSFUNCTIONS IN NEUROENDOCRINE REGULATION WITH IMPLICATIONS TO METABOLIC DISORDERS IN HUMANS

Although it is a widely held thought that direct hormone action on peripheral tissues is sufficient to mediate the control of nutrient handling, the role of the central nervous system in certain aspects of metabolism has long been recognized. Furthermore, recent findings have suggested a more general role for the central nervous system in metabolic control, and have revealed the importance of a number of cues and hypothalamic circuits (Myers & Olson, 2012). The brain's contributions to metabolic control are more readily revealed and the crucial role of neurohormones secreted by cells located in the brain is being confirmed. Over the past decade, numerous reports have underscored the similarities between the metabolism of insects and vertebrates, with the identification of evolutionarily conserved enzymes and analogous organs that regulate carbohydrate and lipid metabolism. It is now well established that the major metabolic, energy-sensing and endocrine signaling networks are also conserved from insects to vertebrates. Accordingly, studies in *Drosophila* are beginning to unravel how perturbed energy balance impinges on lifespan and on the ensuing diseases when energy homeostasis goes awry. Moreover, numerous neurobiological and physiological mechanisms that regulate energy balance exist. In particular, it has become increasingly evident that the brain plays an important role in sensing energy demands and storage in order to maintain/defend body weight within a rather tight range. Studies ranging from worms, flies and mice to humans have identified key conserved genes and neuroal pathways that are critical in regulating energy balance and glucose homeostasis. Since molecular mechanisms for regulation of energy homeostasis in flies and humans are remarkably conserved, investigations of this kind may hold promise for development of novel therapies for metabolic disorders such as diabetes or obesity but also for neurodegenerative diseases such as e.g., Parkinsonians disorders in humans.

DISCLOSURES

The authors declare no competing financial or other conflict of interest.

ACKNOWLEDGMENTS

AB acknowledges Fellowship reg. no. L200961701 from the Programme of Support of Promising Human Resources, awarded by The Czech Academy of Sciences. This research was supported by the start-up funds from Mississippi State University No. 269110-151250 from NSF EPSCOR (NK), by grant No. 14-07172S (DK) from the Czech Science Foundation, and by projects RVO 60077344 of the Institute of Entomology.

REFERENCES

Aarts, E., van Holstein, M., Cools, R. (2011). Striatal dopamine and the interface between motivation and cognition. *Front. Psychol.* 2: article 163.
Abercrombie, E.D., Keefe, K.A., DiFrischia, D.S., Zigmond, M.J. (1989). Differential effect of stress on *in vivo* dopamine release in striatum, nucleus accumbens, and medial frontal cortex. *J. Neurochem.* 52: 1655-1658.

Alic, N., Andrews, T.D, Giannakou, M.E, Papatheodorou, I., Slack, C., Hoddinott, M.P, Cochemé, H.M., Schuster, E.F., Thornton, J.M., Partridge, L. (2011). Genome-wide dFOXO targets and topology of the transcriptomic response to stress and insulin signalling. *Mol. Syst. Biol.* 7: article 502.

Al Saud, S.N., Summerfield, A.C., Alic, N. (2015). Ablation of insulin-producing cells prevents obesity but not premature mortality caused by a high-sugar diet in *Drosophila*. *Proc. Biol. Sci.* 282: article 20141720.

Andretic, R., van Swinderen, B., Greenspan, R.J. (2005). Dopaminergic modulation of arousal in *Drosophila*. *Curr. Biol.* 15: 1165-1175.

Antonova, Y., Arik, A. J., Moore, W., Riehle, M.R., Brown, M.R. (2012). *Insulin-like peptides: structure, signaling, and function.* In: Gilbert L.I. (Ed.), Insect Endocrinology, Elsevier/Academic Press, New York, pp. 63-92.

Argue, K.J., Neckameyer, W.S. (2013). Sexually dimorphic recruitment of dopamine neurons into stress response circuitry. *Behav. Neurosci.* 127: 734-743.

Arquier, N., Bourouis, M., Colombani, J., and Leopold, P. (2005). *Drosophila* Lk6 kinase controls phosphorylation of eukaryotic translation initiation factor 4E and promotes normal growth and development. *Curr. Biol.* 15: 19–23.

Avruch, J., Lin, Y., Long, X., Murthy, S., Ortiz-Vega, S. (2005). Recent advances in the regulation of the TOR pathway by insulin and nutrients. *Curr. Opin. Clin. Nutr. Metab. Care* 8: 67–72.

Bai, H., Kang, P., Tatar, M. (2012). *Drosophila* insulin-like peptide-6 (dilp6) expression from fat body extends lifespan and represses secretion of *Drosophila* insulin-like peptide-2 from the brain. *Aging Cell* 11: 978-985.

Baker, K.D., Thummel, C.S. (2007). Diabetic larvae and obese flies – emerging studies of metabolism in *Drosophila*. *Cell Metab.* 6: 257–266.

Barron, A.B., Søvik E., Cornish, J.L. (2010). The roles of dopamine and related compounds in reward-seeking behavior across animal phyla. *Front. Behav. Neurosci.* 4: article 163.

Bauer, DuMont, V.L., Flores, H.A., Wright, M.H., Aquadro, C.F. (2007). Recurrent positive selection at bgcn, a key determinant of germ line differentiation, does not appear to be driven by simple coevolution with its partner protein bam. *Mol. Biol. Evol.* 24: 182-191.

Bednářová, A., Kodrík, D., Krishnan, N. (2013). Unique roles of glucagon and glucagon-like peptides: Parallels in understanding the functions of adipokinetic hormones in stress responses in insects. *Comp. Biochem. Physiol. Part A.* 164: 91-100.

Bednářová, A., Kodrík, D., Krishnan, N. (2015). Knockdown of adipokinetic hormone synthesis increases susceptibility to oxidative stress in *Drosophila*-a role for dFoxO? *Comp. Biochem. Physiol. Part C* 171: 8-14.

Bednářová, A., Hanna, M.E., Rakshit, K., O'Donnell, J.M., Krishnan, N. (2017). Disruption of dopamine homeostasis has sexually dimorphic effects on senescence characteristics of *Drosophila melanogaster*. *Eur. J. Neurosci.* DOI: 10.1111/ejn.13525

Belmont, M., Cazzamali, G., Williamson, M., Hauser, F., Grimmelikhuijzen, C.J.P. (2006). Identification of four evolutionarily related G protein-coupled receptors from the malaria mosquito *Anopheles gambiae*. *Biochem. Bioph. Res. Co.* 344: 160–165

Bharucha, K.N., Tarr, P, Zipursky, S.L. (2008). A glucagon-like endocrine pathway in *Drosophila* modulates both lipid and carbohydrate homeostasis. *J. Exp. Biol.* 211: 3103-3110.

Bodláková, K., Jedlička, P., Kodrík, D. (2017). Adipokinetic hormones control amylase activity in the cockroach (*Periplaneta americana*) gut. *Insect Sci.* DOI: 10.1111/1744-7917.12314.

Bogomolova, E.V., Rauschenbach, I.Y., Adonyeva, N.V., Alekseev, A.A., Faddeeva, N.V., Gruntenko, N.E. (2010). Dopamine down-regulates activity of alkaline phosphatase in *Drosophila*: the role of D2-Like receptors. *J. Insect Physiol.* 56: 1155-1159.

Botella, J.A, Bayersdorfer, F., Schneuwly, S. (2008). Superoxide dismutase overexpression protects dopaminergic neurons in a *Drosophila* model of Parkinson's disease. *Neurobiol. Dis.* 30: 65-73.

Braco, J.T., Gillespie, E.L., Alberto, G.E., Brenman, J.E., Johnson, E.C. (2012). Energy-dependent modulation of glucagon-like signaling in *Drosophila* via the AMP-activated protein kinase. *Genetics* 192: 457-66.

Britton, J.S., Lockwood, W.K., Li, L., Cohen, S.M., Edgar, B.A. (2002). *Drosophila*'s Insulin/PI3-Kinase pathway coordinates cellular metabolism with nutritional conditions. *Dev. Cell* 2: 239-249.

Brogiolo, W., Stocker, H, Ikeya, T., Rintelen, F., Fernandez, R., Hafen, E. (2001). *An evolutionarily conserved function of the Drosophila insulin receptor and insulin-like peptides in growth control. Curr. Biol.* 11: 213-221.

Broughton, S.J., Piper, M.D., Ikeya, T., Bass, T.M., Jacobson, J., Driege, Y., Martinez, P., Hafen, E., Withers, D.J., Leevers, S.J., Partridge, L. (2005). Longer lifespan, altered metabolism, and stress resistance in *Drosophila* from ablation of cells making insulin-like ligands. *Proc. Natl. Acad. Sci. USA.* 102: 3105-3110.

Brunet, A., Bonni, A., Zigmond, M.J., Lin, M.Z., Juo, P., Hu, L.S., Anderson, M.J., Arden, K.C., Blenis, J., Greenberg, M.E. (1999). Akt promotes cell survival by phosphorylating and inhibiting a Forkhead transcription factor. *Cell* 96: 857-868.

Buch, S., Melcher, C., Bauer, M., Katzenberger, J., Pankratz, M.J. (2008). Opposing effects of dietary protein and sugar regulate a transcriptional target of *Drosophila* insulin-like peptide signaling. *Cell Metab.* 7: 321-332.

Burt, J., Dube, L., Thibault, L., Gruber, R. (2014). Sleep and eating in childhood: a potential behavioral mechanism underlying the relationship between poor sleep and obesity. *Sleep Med.* 15: 71–75.

Cagniard, B, Beeler, J.A, Britt, J.P., McGehee, D.S., Marinelli, M., Zhuang X. (2006). Dopamine scales performance in the absence of new learning. *Neuron.* 51: 541–547.

Cao, C., Brown, M.R. (2001). *Localization of an insulin-like peptide in brains of two flies. Cell Tissue Res.* 304: 317–321.

Chaudhuri, A., Bowling, K., Funderburk, C., Lawal, H., Inamdar, A., Wang, Z., O'Donnell, J.M. (2007). Interaction of genetic and environmental factors in a *Drosophila* Parkinsonism model. *J. Neurosci.* 27: 2457-2467.

Colombani, J., Andersen, D.S., Leopold, P. (2012). *Secreted peptide Dilp8 coordinates Drosophila tissue growth with developmental timing.* Science 336: 582-585.

Colombani, J., Raisin, S., Pantalacci, S., Radimerski, T., Montagne, J., Léopold, P. (2003). A nutrient sensor mechanism controls *Drosophila* growth. *Cell* 114: 739-749.

Cognigni, P., Bailey, A.P., Miguel-Aliaga, I. (2011). *Enteric neurons and systemic signals couple nutritional and reproductive status with intestinal homeostasis.* Cell Metab. 13: 92-104.

D'Angio, M., Serrano, A., Driscoll, P., Scatton, B. (1988). Stressful environmental stimuli increase extracellular DOPAC levels in the prefrontal cortex of hypoemotional (Roman high-avoidance) but not hyperemotional (Roman low-avoidance) rats. An *in vivo* voltametric study. *Brain Res.* 451: 237-247.

Dann, S. G., Thomas, G. (2006). The amino acid sensitive TOR pathway from yeast to mammals. *FEBS Lett.* 580: 2821-2829.

Davenport, A.P, Evans, P.D. (1984). Stress-induced changes in the octopamine levels of insect haemolymph. *Insect Biochem.* 14: 135-143.

Demontis, F., Perrimon, N. (2010). FOXO/4E-BP signaling in *Drosophila* muscles regulates organism-wide proteostasis during aging. *Cell* 143: 813–825.

DiAngelo, J.R., Birnbaum, M.J. (2009). Regulation of fat cell mass by insulin in *Drosophila* melanogaster. *Mol. Cell. Biol.* 29: 6341-6352.

Dobson, A.J., Ezcurra, M., Flanagan, C.E., Summerfield, A.C., Piper, M.D.W., Gems, D., Alic, N. (2017). Nutritional programming of lifespan by FOXO inhibition on sugar-rich diets. *Cell Rep.* 18: 299-582.

Drucker, D.J., Philippe, J, Mojsov, S, Chick, W.L., Habener, J.F. (1987). Glucagon-likepeptide I stimulates insulin gene expression and increases cyclic AMP levels in a rat islet cell line. *Pro. Natl. Acad. Sci. USA* 84: 3434-3438.

Edgar, B.A. (2006). How flies get their size: genetics meets physiology. *Nat. Rev. Genet.* 7: 907–916.

Enell, L.E., Kapan, N, Söderberg, J.A., Kahsai, L, Nässel, D.R. (2010). Insulin signaling, lifespan and stress resistance are modulated by metabotropic GABA receptors on insulin producing cells in the brain of *Drosophila*. *PLoS One* 5: e1578.

Essers, M.A., Weijzen, S., de Vries-Smits, A.M., Saarloos, I., de Ruiter, N.D., Bos, J.L., Burgering, B.M. (2004). FOXO transcription factor activation by oxidative stress mediated by the small GTPase Ral and JNK. *EMBO J.* 23: 4802-4812.

Fabrizio, P., Pozza, F., Pletcher, S.D., Gendron, C.M., Longo, V.D. (2001). Regulation of longevity and stress resistance by Sch9 in yeast. *Science* 292: 288-290.

Fairburn, C.G., Harrison, P.J. (2003). Eating disorders. *Lancet* 361: 407-416.

Fernandez, R., Tabarini, D., Azpiazu, N., Frasch, M., Schlessinger, J. (1995). The *Drosophila* insulin receptor homolog: a gene essential for embryonic development encodes two receptor isoforms with different signaling potential. *EMBO J.* 14: 3373-3384.

Figlewicz, D.P., Szot, P., Chavez, M., Woods, S.C., Veith, R.C. (1994). Intraventricular insulin increases dopamine transporter mRNA in rat VTA/substantia nigra. *Brain Res.* 644: 331-334.

Fontana, L., Partridge, L., Longo, V.D. (2010). Extending healthy life span–from yeast to humans. *Science* 328: 321-326.

Gáliková, M., Diesner, M., Klepsatel, P., Hehlert, P., Xu, Y., Bickmeyer, I., Predel, R., Kühnlein, R.P. (2015). Energy homeostasis control in *Drosophila* adipokinetic hormone mutants. *Genetics* 201: 665-683.

Gáliková, M., Klepsatel, P., Xu, Y., Kühnlein, R.P. (2016). The obesity-related adipokinetic hormone controls feeding and expression of neuropeptide regulators of *Drosophila* metabolism. *Eur. J. Lipid Sci. Technol.* doi:10.1002/ejlt.201600138.

Gäde, G., Hoffmann, K.H., Spring, J.H. (1997). Hormonal regulation in insects: facts, gaps, and future directions. *Physiol. Rev.* 77: 963-1032.

Gao, Q., Horvath, T.L. (2008). Neuronal control of energy homeostasis. *FEBS Lett.* 582: 132-141.

Garelli, A., Gontijo, A.M., Miguela, V., Caparros, E., Dominguez, M. (2012). Imaginal discs secrete insulin-like peptide 8 to mediate plasticity of growth and maturation. *Science* 336: 579-582.

Garofalo, R.S. (2002). Genetic analysis of insulin signaling in Drosophila. *Trends Endocrin. Met.* 13: 156-162.

Geminard, G., Arquier, N., Layalle, S., Bourouis, M., Slaidina, M., Delanoue, R., Bjordal, M., Ohanna, M., Ma, M., Colombani, J., Léopold, P. (2006). Control of metabolism and growth through insulin-like peptides in Drosophila. *Diabetes* 55: S5-S8.

Géminard, C., Rulifson, E.J., Léopold, P. (2009). Remote control of insulin secretion by fat cells in Drosophila. *Cell Metab.* 10: 199-207.

Giannakou, M.E., Partridge, L. (2007). Role of insulin-like signalling in *Drosophila* lifespan. *Trends Biochem Sci* 32: 180-188.

Giannakou, M.E., Goss, M., Partridge, L. (2008). Role of dFOXO in lifespan extension by dietary restriction in *Drosophila melanogaster*: not required, but its activity modulates the response. *Aging Cell* 7: 187-198.

Glauser, D.A., Schelegel, W. (2007). The emerging role of FOXO transcription factors in pancreatic beta cells. *J. Endocrinol.* 193: 195-207.

Greer, C.L., Grygoruk, A., Patton, D.E., Ley, B., Romero-Calderon, R., Chang, H.Y., Houshyar, R., Bainton, R.J., Diantonio, A., Krantz, D.E. (2005). A splice variant of the *Drosophila* vesicular monoamine transporter contains a conserved trafficking domain and functions in the storage of dopamine, serotonin, and octopamine. *J. Neurobiol.* 64: 239-258.

Grönke, S., Clarke, D. F., Broughton, S., Andrews, T.D., Partridge, L. (2010). Molecular evolution and functional characterization of Drosophila insulin-like peptides. *PLoS Genet.* 6, e1000857.

Gruntenko, N.E., Adonyeva, N.V., Burdina, E.V., Karpova, E.K., Andreenkova, O.V., Gladkikh, D.V., Ilinsky, Y.Y., Rauschenbach, I.Y. (2016). The impact of FOXO on dopamine and octopamine metabolism in *Drosophila* under normal and heat stress conditions. *Biol. Open.* 5: 1706-1711.

Guertin, D.A., Sabatini, D.M. (2007). Defining the role of mTOR in cancer. *Cancer Cell.* 12: 9-22.

Hafen, E. (2004). Interplay between growth factor and nutrient signaling: Lessons from *Drosophila* TOR. *Curr. Top. Microbiol. Immunol.* 279: 153-167.

Hald, A, Lotharius, J. (2005). Oxidative stress and inflammation in Parkinson's disease: is there a causal link? *Exp. Neurol.* 193: 279-290.

Hanna, M.E., Bednářová, A., Rakshit, K., Chaudhuri, A., O'Donnell, J.M., Krishnan, N. (2015). Perturbations in dopamine synthesis lead to discrete physiological effects and impact oxidative stress response in Drosophila. *J. Insect Physiol.* 73: 11-19.

Hansen, K.K., Stafflinger, E., Schneider, M., Hauser, F., Cazzamali, G., Williamson, M., Kollmann M., Schachtner, J., Grimmelikhuijzen, C.J.P. (2010). Discovery of a novel insect neuropeptide signaling system closely related to the insect adipokinetic hormone and corazonin hormonal systems. *J. Biol. Chem.* 285: 10736-10747.

Hauser, F., Sondergaard, L., Grimmelikhuijzen, C.J.P. (1998). Molecular cloning, genomic organization and developmental regulation of a novel receptor from *Drosophila melanogaster* structurally related to gonadotropin-releasing hormone receptors from vertebrates. *Biochem. Bioph. Res. Co.* 249: 822-828.

Hay, N., Sonenberg, N. (2004). Upstream and downstream of mTOR. *Gen. Dev.* 18: 1926-1945.

Hirosumi, J., Tuncman, G., Chang, L., Görgün, C.Z., Uysal, K.T., Maeda, K., Karin, M., Hotamisligil, G.S. (2002). A central role for JNK in obesity and insulin resistance. *Nature* 420: 333-336.

Hnasko, T.S., Szczypka, M.S., Alaynick, W.A., During, M.J., Palmiter, R.D. (2004). A role for dopamine in feeding responses produced by orexigenic agents. *Brain Res.* 1023: 309-318.

Hoebel, B.G. (1971). Feeding: neural control of intake. *Annu. Rev. Physiol.* 33: 533-568.

Hotamisligil, G.S. (2006). Inflammation and metabolic disorders. *Nature* 444: 860-867.

Hsouna, A., Lawal, H.O., Izevbaye, I., Hsu, T., O'Donnell, J.M. (2007). *Drosophila* dopamine synthesis pathway genes regulate tracheal morphogenesis. *Dev. Biol.* 308: 30-43.

Hwangbo, D.S., Gersham, B., Tu, M.P., Palmer, M., Tatar, M. (2004). *Drosophila* dFOXO controls lifespan and regulates insulin signalling in brain and fat body. *Nature* 429: 562-566.

Hyman, S.E., Cole R.L., Konradi, C., Kosofsky, B.E. (1995). Dopamine regulation of transcription factor-target interactions in rat striatum. *Chemical Senses* 20: 257-260.

Ikeya, T., Galic M., Belawat, P., Nairz, K., Hafen, E. (2002). Nutrient-dependent expression of insulin-like peptides from neuroendocrine cells in the CNS contributes to growth regulation in *Drosophila*. *Curr. Biol.* 12: 1293-300.

Isabel, G., Martin, J.R., Chidami, S., Veenstra, J.A., Rosay P. (2005). AKH-producing neuroendocrine cell ablation decreases trehalose and induces behavioral changes in *Drosophila*. *Am. J. Physiol. Regul. Integr. Comp. Physiol.* 288: 531-538.

Johnson, E.C., White, M.P. (2009). "Stressed-out insects: hormonal actions and behavioral modifications". In: Pfaff D.W., Arnold A.P., Etgen A.M., Fahrbach S.E., Rubin R.T. (Eds.), *Hormones, Brain and Behavior*, Elsevier Academic Press, San Diego, pp 1069-1096.

Jünger, M.A., Rintelen, F., Stocker, H., Wasserman, J.D., Végh, M., Radimerski, T., Greenberg, M.E., Hafen, E. (2003). The *Drosophila* forkhead transcription factor FOXO mediates the reduction in cell number associated with reduced insulin signaling, *J. Biol.* 2, 20.

Kabil, H., Partridge, L., Harshman, L.G. (2007). Superoxide dismutase activities in long-lived *Drosophila melanogaster* females: chico1 genotypes and dietary dilution. *Biogerontology* 8: 201-208.

Karpac, J., Jasper, H. (2009). Insulin and JNK: optimizing metabolic homeostasis and lifespan. *Trends Endocrin. Met.* 20: 100-106.

Kim, S.K., Rulifson, E.J. (2004). Conserved mechanisms of glucose sensing and regulation by *Drosophila* corpora cardiaca cells. *Nature* 431:316-320.

Kodrík, D. (2008). Adipokinetic hormone functions that are not associated with insect flight. *Physiol. Entomol.* 33: 171-180.

Kodrík, D., Krishnan, N., Habuštová, O. (2007). Is the titer of adipokinetic peptides in *Leptinotarsa decemlineata* fed on genetically modified potatoes increased by oxidative stress? *Peptides* 28: 974-980.

Kodrík, D., Bednářová, A., Zemanová, M., Krishnan, N. (2015). Hormonal Regulation of Response to Oxidative Stress in Insects-An Update. *Int. J. Mol. Sci.* 16: 25788-25816.

Kodrík, D., Vinokurov, K., Tomčala, A., Socha, R. (2012). The effect of adipokinetic hormone on midgut characteristics in *Pyrrhocoris apterus* L. (Heteroptera). *J. Insect Physiol.* 58: 194-204.

Kodrík, D., Socha, R., Šimek, P., Zemek, R., Goldsworthy, G.J. (2000). A new member of the AKH/RPCH family that stimulates locomotory activity in the firebug, *Pyrrhocoris apterus* (Heteroptera), *Insect Biochem. Mol. Biol.* 30: 489-498.

Kodrík, D., Stašková, T., Jedličková, V., Weyda, F., Závodská, R., Pflegerová, J. (2015). Molecular characterization, tissue distribution, and ultrastructural localization of adipokinetic hormones in the CNS of the firebug *Pyrrhocoris apterus* (Heteroptera, Insecta). *Gen. Comp. Endocrinol.* 210: 1-11.

Kramer, J.M., Slade, J.D., Staveley, B.E. (2008). Foxo is required for resistance to amino acid starvation in *Drosophila*. *Genome* 51: 668-672.

Kreneisz, O, Chen, X, Fridell, Y.W., Mulkey, D.K. (2010). Glucose increases activity and Ca($^{2+}$) in insulin-producing cells of adult *Drosophila*. *Neuroreport* 21: 1116–1120.

Krishnan, N., Kodrík, D. (2012). Endocrine control of oxidative stress in insects. In: Farooqui T. and Farooqui A. A. (Eds.), *Oxidative Stress in Vertebrates and Invertebrates: Molecular Aspects of Oxidative Stress on Cell Signaling,* Wiley-Blackwell, New Jersey, pp *261-270*.

Kume, K., Kume, S., Park, S.K., Hirsh, J., Jackson, F.R. (2005). Dopamine is a regulator of arousal in the fruit fly. *J. Neurosci.* 25: 7377-7384.

Lee, G., Park, J.H. (2004). Hemolymph sugar homeostasis and starvation-induced hyperactivity affected by genetic manipulations of the adipokinetic hormone-encoding gene in *Drosophila melanogaster*. *Genetics* 167: 311-323.

Lee, K.S., Kwon, O.Y., Lee, J.H., Kwon, K, Min, K.J., Jung, S.A., Kim, A.K., You, K.H., Tatar, M., Yu, K. (2008). Drosophila short neuropeptide F signaling regulates growth by ERK-mediated insulin signaling. *Nat. Cell Biol.* 10: 468-475.

Li, S., Hauser, F., Skadborg, S.K., Nielsen, S.V., Kirketerp-Møller, N., Grimmelikhuijzen S.J.P. (2016). Adipokinetic hormones and their G protein-coupled receptors emerged in Lophotrochozoa. *Sci. Rep.* 6: article 32789.

Linneweber, G. A., Jacobson, J., Busch, K.E., Hudry, B., Christov, C.P., Dormann, D., Yuan, M., Otani, T., Knust, E., de Bono, M., Miguel-Aliaga, I. (2014). *Neuronal control of metabolism through nutrient-dependent modulation of tracheal branching.* Cell 156: 69–83.

Lopez-Maury, L., Marguerat, S. Bahler, J. (2008). Tuning gene expression to changing environments: from rapid responses to evolutionary adaptation. *Nat. Rev. Genet.* 9: 583-593.

Martin, C.A, Krantz, D.E. (2014). *Drosophila melanogaster* as a genetic model system to study neurotransmitter transporters. *Neurochem. Int.* 73: 71-88.

Mebel, D.M., Wong, J.C.Y., Dong, Y.J., Bogland, S.L. (2012). Insulin in the ventral tegmental area reduces hedonic feeding and suppresses dopamine concentration via increased uptake. *Eur. J. Neurosci.* 36: 2236-2246.

Meissner, G.W., Luo, S.D., Dias, B.G., Texada, M.J. Baker, B.S. (2016). Sex-specific regulation of Lgr3 in Drosophila neurons. *Proc. Natl. Acad. Sci. USA* 113: 1256-1265.

Miguel-Aliaga, I., Thor, S., Gould, A.P. (2008). Postmitotic specification of Drosophila insulinergic neurons from pioneer neurons. *PLoS Biol.* 6, e58.

Mirth, C.K., Tang, H.Y., Makohon-Moore, S.C., Salhadar, S., Gokhale, R.H., Warner, R.D., Koyama, T., Riddiford, L.M. and Shingleton, A.W. (2014). Juvenile hormone regulates body size and perturbs insulin signaling in *Drosophila*. *Proc. Natl. Acad. Sci. USA* 111: 7018-7023.

Münzberg, H., Qualls-Creekmore, E., Berthoud, H.R., Morrison, C.D., Yu, S. (2016). Neural control of energy expenditure. *Handb. Exp. Pharmacol.* 233: 173-194.
Myers, M.G, Jr., Olson, D.P. (2012). Central nervous system control of metabolism. *Nature* 491: 357-363.
Nässel, D. R., Kubrak, O. I., Liu, Y., Luo, J., Lushchak, O. V. (2013). Factors that regulate insulin producing cells and their output in Drosophila. *Front. Physiol.* 4: article 252.
Neckameyer, W.S. (1996). Multiple roles for dopamine in *Drosophila* development. *Dev. Biol.* 176: 209-219.
Neckameyer, W.S., White, K. (1993). *Drosophila* tyrosine hydroxylase is encoded by the pale locus. *J. Neurogenet.* 8: 189-199.
Neckameyer, W.S., Woodrome, S., Holt, B., Mayer, A. (2000). Dopamine and senescence in *Drosophila melanogaster*. *Neurobiol. Aging* 21: 145-152.
Oh, S.W., Mukhopadhyay, A., Svrzikapa, N., Jiang, F., Davis, R.J. Tissenbaum, H.A. (2005). JNK regulates lifespan in Caenorhabditis elegans by modulating nuclear translocation of forkhead transcription factor/DAF-16. *Proc. Natl. Acad. Sci. USA*, 102: 4494-4499.
Okamoto, N. Yamanaka, N., Yagi, Y., Nishida, Y., Kataoka, H., O'Connor, M.B., Mizoguchi, A. (2009). A fat body-derived IGF-like peptide regulates postfeeding growth in *Drosophila*. *Dev. Cell* 17: 885-891.
Owusu-Ansah, E., Perrimon, N. (2014). Modeling metabolic homeostasis and nutrient sensing in *Drosophila*: implications for aging and metabolic diseases. *Dis. Model. Mech.* 7: 343-350.
Padmanabha, D., Baker, K.D. (2014). *Drosophila* gains traction as a repurposed tool to investigate metabolism. *Trends Endocrin. Met.* 25: 489-554.
Palmiter, R.D. (2007). Is dopamine a physiologically relevant mediator of feeding behavior? *Trends Neurosci.* 30: 375-381.
Park, S., Alfa R.W., Topper, S.M, Kim, G.E., Kockel L., Kim S.K. (2014). A genetic strategy to measure circulating *Drosophila* insulin reveals genes regulating insulin production and secretion. *PLoS Genet.* 10: e1004555.

Pendleton, R.G., Rasheed, A., Sardina, T., Tully, T., Hillman, R. (2002). Effects of tyrosine hydroxylase mutants on locomotor activity in *Drosophila*: a study in functional genomics. *Behav. Genet.* 32: 89-94.

Perić-Mataruga, V., Nenadović, V., Ivanović, J. (2006). Neurohormones in insect stress: A review. *Arch. Biol. Sci. Belgrade* 58: 1-12.

Post, S., Tatar, M. (2016). Nutritional Geometric Profiles of Insulin/IGF Expression in *Drosophila melanogaster*. *PLoS One* 11: e0155628.

Puig, O., Marr, M.T., Ruhf, M.L., Tjian, R. (2003). Control of cell number by *Drosophila* FOXO: Downstream and feedback regulation of the insulin receptor pathway. *Gen. Dev.* 17: 2006-2020.

Rauschenbach, I.Y., Karpova, E.K., Gruntenko, N.E. (2015). dFOXO transcription factor regulates juvenile hormone metabolism in *Drosophila melanogaster* females. *Rus. J. Genet.* 51: 932-934.

Rauschenbach, I.Y., Karpova, E.K., Adonyeva, N.V., Andreenkova, O.V., Faddeeva, N.V., Burdina, E.V., Alekseev, A.A., Menshanov, P.N., Gruntenko, N.E. (2014). Disruption of insulin signalling affects the neuroendocrine stress reaction in *Drosophila* females. *J. Exp. Biol.* 217: 3733-3741.

Rajan, A., Perrimon, N. (2012). *Drosophila* cytokine unpaired 2 regulates physiological homeostasis by remotely controlling insulin secretion. *Cell* 151: 123-37.

Reiling, J.H., Doepfner, K.T., Hafen, E., Stocker, H. (2005). Diet-dependent effects of the *Drosophila* Mnk1/Mnk2 homolog Lk6 on growth via eIF4E. *Curr. Biol.* 15: 24-30.

Rulifson, E.J., Kim, S.K., Nusse, R. (2002). Ablation of insulin-producing neurons in flies: growth and diabetic phenotypes. *Science* 296: 1118–1120.

Russell, S.J., Kahn, C.R. (2007). Endocrine regulation of ageing. *Nat. Rev. Mol. Cell Biol.* 8: 681-691.

Sabban, E.L. 2007. Catecholamines in stress: molecular mechanisms of gene expression. *Endocr. Regul.* 41: 61-73.

Sajwan, S., Sidorov, R., Stašková, T., Žaloudíková, A., Takasu, Y., Kodrík, D., Zurovec, M. (2015). Targeted mutagenesis and functional analysis of adipokinetic hormone-encoding gene in *Drosophila*. *Insect Biochem. Mol. Biol.* 61: 79-86.

Sano, H., Nakamura, A., Texada, M.J., Truman, J.W., Ishimoto, H., Kamikouchi, A., Nibu, Y., Kume, K., Ida, T., Kojima, M. (2015). The nutrient-responsive hormone cchamide-2 controls growth by regulating insulin-like peptides in the brain of *Drosophila melanogaster*. *PLoS Genet.* 11: e1005209.

Schultz, W. (2006). Behavioral theories and the neurophysiology of reward. *Annu. Rev. Psychol.* 57: 87-115.

Schumacher, B., Garinis, G.A., Hoeijmakers, J.H.J. (2008). Age to survive: DNA damage and aging. *Trends Genet.* 24: 77-85.

Shi, Y., Huang, H., Deng, X., He, X., Yang, J., Yang, H., Shi, L., Mei, L., Gao, J., Zhou, N. (2011). Identification and functional characterization of two orphan G-protein-coupled receptors for adipokinetic hormones from silkworm *Bombyx mori*. *J. Biol. Chem.* 286: 42390-42402.

Slade, J.D., Staveley, B.E. (2016). Manipulation of components that control feeding behavior in *Drosophila melanogaster* increases sensitivity to amino acid starvation. *Genet. Mol. Res.* 15: article gmr.15017489.

Slaidina, M., Delanoue, R., Grönke, S., Partridge, L., Leopold, P. (2009). A *Drosophila* insulin-like peptide promotes growth during nonfeeding states. *Dev. Cell* 17: 874-884.

Socha, R., Kodrík, D., Zemek, R. (1999). Stimulation of locomotion in *Pyrrhocoris apterus* (Heteroptera: Pyrrhocoridae) is wing-morph independent and correlated with lipid mobilization by adipokinetic hormone, *Eur. J. Entomol.* 96: 459-461.

Söderberg, J.A.E., Birse, R.T., Nässel, D.R. (2011). Insulin production and signaling in renal tubules of *Drosophila* is under control of tachykinin-related peptide and regulates stress resistance. *PLoS One* 6: e19866.

Söderberg, J. A., Carlsson, M. A., Nässel, D.R. (2012). Insulin-producing cells in the *Drosophila* brain also express satiety-inducing cholecystokinin-like peptide, drosulfakinin. *Front. Endocrinol.* 3: 109.

Sonoda, N., Imamura, T., Yoshizaki, T., Babendure, J.L., Lu, J.C., Olefsky, J.M. (2008). Beta-arrestin-1 mediates glucagon-like peptide-1 signaling to insulin secretion in cultured pancreatic beta cells. *Proc. Natl. Acad. Sci. USA* 105: 6614-6619.

Sotak, B.N., Hnasko, T.S., Robinson, S., Kremer, E.J., Palmiter, R.D. (2005). Dysregulation of dopamine signaling in the dorsal striatum inhibits feeding. *Brain Res.* 1061: 88-96.

Speed, N., Saunders, C., Davis, A.R., Owens, W.A., Matthies, H.J., Saadat, S., Kennedy, J.P., Vaughan, R.A., Neve, R.L., Lindsley, C.W., Russo, S.J., Daws, L.C., Niswender, K.D., Galli, A. (2011). Impaired striatal Akt signaling disrupts dopamine homeostasis and increases feeding. *PLoS One* 6: e25169.

Spellberg, M.J., Marr, M.T. (2015). FOXO regulates RNA interference in *Drosophila* and protects from RNA virus infection. *Proc. Natl. Acad. Sci. USA* 112: 14587-14592.

Stathakis, D.G., Burton, D.Y., McIvor, W.E., Krishnakumar, S., Wright, T.R., O'Donnell, J.M. (1999). The catecholamines up (Catsup) protein of *Drosophila melanogaster* functions as a negative regulator of tyrosine hydroxylase activity. *Genetics* 153: 361-382.

Staubli, F., Jorgensen, T.J., Cazzamali, G., Williamson, M., Lenz, C., Sondergaard, L., Roepstorff, P., Grimmelikhuijzen C.J. (2002). Molecular identification of the insect adipokinetic hormone receptors. *Proc. Natl. Acad. Sci. USA* 99: 3446-3451.

Stone, J.V., Mordue, W., Batley, K.E., Morris, H.R. (1976). Structure of locust adipokinetic hormone, a neurohormone that regulates lipid utilisation during flight. *Nature* 263: 207-221.

Szczypka, M.S., Rainey, M.A., Kim, D.S., Alaynick W.A., Marck B.T., Matsumoto A.M., Palmiter R.D. (1999). Feeding behavior in dopamine-deficient mice. *Proc. Natl. Acad. Sci. USA* 96: 12138-12143.

Taguchi, A., White, M.F. (2008). Insulin-like signaling, nutrient homeostasis, and life span. *Annu. Rev. Physiol.* 70: 191-212.

Tatar, M., Yin, C. (2001). Slow aging during insect reproductive diapause: why butterflies, grasshoppers and flies are like worms. *Exp. Gerontol.* 36: 723-738.

Tatar, M., Bartke, A., Antebi, A. (2003). The endocrine regulation of aging by insulin-like signals. *Science* 299: 1346-51.

Teleman, A.A. (2010). Molecular mechanisms of metabolic regulation by insulin in *Drosophila*. *Biochem. J.* 425: 13-26.

Teleman, A.A., Chen, Y.W., Cohen, S.M. (2005). *Drosophila* melted modulates FOXO and TOR activity. *Dev. Cell* 9: 271-281.

Tettweiler, G., Miron, M., Jenkins, M., Sonenberg, N., Lasko, P.F. (2005). Starvation and oxidative stress resistance in *Drosophila* are mediated through the eIF4E-binding protein, d4E-BP. *Gen. Dev.* 19: 1840-1843.

Toivonen, J. M., Partridge, L. (2009). Endocrine regulation of aging and reproduction in *Drosophila*. *Mol. Cell. Endocrinol.* 299: 39-50.

Unger, R.H., Cherrington, A.D. (2012). Glucagonocentric restructuring of diabetes: a pathophysiologic and therapeutic makeover. *J. Clin. Invest.* 122: 4-12.

Wang, M.C., Bohmann, D., Jasper, H. (2005). JNK extends life span and limits growth by antagonizing cellular and organism-wide responses to insulin signaling. *Cell* 121: 115-125.

Wang, B., Moya, N., Niessen, S., Hoover, H., Mihaylova, M.M., Shaw, R.J., Yates, J.R., Fischer, W.H., Thomas, J.B., Montminy, M. (2011). A hormone-dependent module regulating energy balance. *Cell* 145: 596-606.

Wise, R.A. (2002). Brain reward circuitry: insights from unsensed incentives. *Neuron* 36: 229-240.

Wolfrum, C., Besser, D., Luca, E., Stoffel, M. (2003). Insulin regulates the activity of forkhead transcription factor Hnf-3β/Foxa-2 by Akt-mediated phosphorylation and nuclear/cytosolic localization. *Proc. Natl. Acad. Sci. USA* 100: 11624–11629.

Wolfrum, C., Asilmaz, E., Luca, E., Friedman, J.M., Stoffel, M. (2004). Foxa2 regulates lipid metabolism and ketogenesis in the liver during fasting and in diabetes. *Nature* 432:1027-1032.

Wu, Q., Brown, M.R. (2006). Signaling and function of insulin-like peptides in insects. *Annu. Rev. Entomol.* 51: 1-24.

Wullschleger, S., Loewith, R., Hall, M.N. (2006). TOR signaling in growth and metabolism. *Cell* 124: 471-84.

Yamamoto, S., Seto, E.S. (2014). Dopamine dynamics and signaling in *Drosophila*: an overview of genes, drugs and behavioral paradigms. *Exp. Anim.* 63: 107-119.

Yamamoto, K., Vernier, P. (2011). The evolution of dopamine systems in chordates. *Front. Neuroanat.* 5: article 21.

Yang, C.H., Belawat, P., Hafen, E., Jan, L.Y., Jan, Y.N. (2008). *Drosophila* egg-laying site selection as a system to study simple decision-making processes. *Science* 319: 1679-1683.

In: Advances in Health and Disease
Editor: Lowell T. Duncan

ISBN: 978-1-53613-020-1
© 2018 Nova Science Publishers, Inc.

Chapter 2

EXPLORING MICRO -, MEZZO -, AND MACRO- LEVEL FACTORS IMPACTING HIV TESTING BEHAVIORS AMONG ASIAN AMERICANS AND PACIFIC ISLANDER

Soma Sen[1,*], PhD, Van Ta Park[2,†], PhD, Malaya Arevalo[3,‡], So Yung Kim[1,§] and Hoang Dung Nguyen[1,#]
[1]School of Social Work, San Jose State University,
San Jose, CA, US
[2]Department of Community Health Systems,
University of California at San Francisco,
San Francisco, CA, US
[3]Department of Wellness Services,
Asian Americans for Community Involvement,
San Jose, CA, US

---

[*] soma.sen@sjsu.edu.
[†] van.park@ucsf.edu.
[‡] Malaya.arevalo@aaci.org.
[§] kimsoyung@gmail.com.
[#] hoang_dung_1120@yahoo.com.

Abstract

Asian Americans and Pacific Islanders (AAPI) are the only racial group in the U.S. with a significant increase in HIV rates and delayed HIV testing. However, factors impacting HIV testing in this population is poorly understood. Hence, this mixed method study examines the various individual, familial, structural factors that impact testing behavior in this population. Findings revealed various barriers to testing including a lack of HIV related knowledge and low perception of risk, a family culture of silence around HIV, HIV related stigma, fear of losing social/sexual networks, and fear of dealing with the diagnosis alone. These findings indicate a necessity to understand the decision making process that impact HIV testing and to design interventions to mitigate the impact of stigma.

Introduction

Asian Americans and Pacific Islanders (AAPI) are among the fastest growing racial and ethnic groups in the United States with an 11% growth rate between 2010 and 2014, more than three times faster than the total U.S. population. During the same period, the number of AAPI receiving an HIV diagnosis also increased by 36%, driven primarily by an increase in HIV diagnoses among AAPI Men who have Sex with Men (Centers for Disease Control and Prevention [CDC], 2014). Such a trend was also detected in the early 2000s. In fact, an analysis of surveillance data from 33 states between 2001 and 2008 showed AAPI to be the group with the highest increase in HIV diagnosis rates of all races/ethnicities (Adih, Campsmith, Williams, Hardnett, & Hughes, 2011). What is particularly concerning about the increase in new HIV diagnosis for the AAPI community is the high number of potentially undiagnosed individuals living with HIV or Acquired Immunodeficiency Syndrome (AIDS). The CDC (2016) reports that 21% of AAPI living with HIV or AIDS in the United States are undiagnosed, compared with 13% of the total U.S. population. This would imply that the current diagnosis rates would likely be much higher than reported. A case in point are the high number of HIV cases in the AAPI community that are initially diagnosed at an advanced stage of the disease (Wong, Campsmith,

Nakamura, Crepaz & Begley, 2004; Zaidi et al., 2005). Approximately 24.6% of new HIV diagnoses among AAPI in 2014 were diagnosed with both AIDS and HIV at the same time (CDC, 2016). Thus at initial diagnosis, AAPI are more likely to have an opportunistic infection or other AIDS-defining characteristics. These data suggest that AAPI are either waiting to be tested or not getting tested at all, which increases concerns about HIV transmission to their sexual partners.

Furthermore, within AAPI communities, certain subgroups such as women, Men who have Sex with Men (MSM) and injection drug users show particular vulnerabilities. The available studies suggest that AAPI are as likely as other racial/ethnic groups to engage in HIV-related risk behaviors, but are less likely than other racial/ethnic groups to have ever tested for HIV (Huang, Wong, De Leon, & Park, 2008; Zaidi et al., 2005).

Studies on risk factors show that transmission for AAPI men is primarily due to male-to-male sexual contact (89%) while for women it is largely due to high-risk heterosexual contact (95%). Available data suggests that AAPI MSM constitute 74% of all cases among AAPI since the beginning of the epidemic and 52% of the new AIDS cases (CDC, 2015). While injection drug use, an important transmission risk for both AAPI men and women are at 4% and 5%, respectively (compared to 6% in the general population), the relationship between substance abuse and HIV-risk behaviors among AAPI has receives little attention. Choi and colleagues (2005) examined drug use among a sample of 496 AAPI MSM and found that 47% reported unprotected anal sex in the past six months and that having unprotected anal sex was associated with being high or "buzzed" on ecstasy and poppers during sex. Operario and Nemoto (2005) found that 13% of their sample of AAPI male-to-female transgender individuals reported being HIV positive and that during a one-month period, 20% had unprotected receptive anal intercourse with men, 49% used non-injection drugs, and 4% injected drugs.

These trends are alarming, to begin with, but become even more significant in the light of underreporting and a lack of existing detailed surveillance data because these issues mask the true nature of the HIV epidemic in this population. While HIV testing is considered an essential component of comprehensive HIV prevention and education efforts (Trieu,

Modeste, Marshak, Males, & Bratton, 2008), research indicate that HIV positive AAPI are less likely to know their current CD4 status, and are less knowledgeable about the availability of HIV-related care services than Whites (Adih et al., 2011).

There are many possible reasons for delayed testing, HIV-related stigma being one of the primary reasons. Many AAPI come from traditional family structures, which frown upon public discussions of sexual activity and view homosexuality as a strictly Western phenomenon (Chin, Leung, Sheth, & Rodriguez, 2007). These cultural beliefs can deter AAPI from testing for HIV while still engaging in unsafe sex practices. In addition, recent AAPI immigrants generally work low-wage jobs and lack access to medical insurance; this impacts infected individuals' ability and motivation to seek medical attention until the disease has reached advanced stages, thus, increasing the likelihood of disease transmission (Chng, Wong, Park, Edberg & Lai, 2003).

Despite the fact that the data presented above indicates a frightening trend in the AAPI communities, there is a limited understanding of HIV-related risk behaviors and HIV testing behaviors among AAPI, as well as the various factors that act as barriers and facilitators to HIV testing among AAPI. This mixed-methods study aimed to add to the existing body of knowledge in this area by exploring the various factors that impact HIV-testing behaviors among AAPI.

LITERATURE REVIEW

HIV testing is a critical first step in diagnosing and linking people with HIV to medical care. The CDC (CDC, 2014) has acknowledged that challenges to HIV prevention in AAPI communities persist. Cultural barriers such as language, homophobia, and maintaining family reputations may also impact AAPI' motivations to seek testing or treatment. Moreover, the U.S. Census (2013) identified the influence of the "model minority" stereotype, i.e., that Asians generally have high educational and economic success and therefore are "problem-free," as prompting researchers to believe that AAPI communities have quality health care and are in good overall health. This has contributed to the limited number of empirical studies on HIV-related subjects among AAPI.

Given that this study aims to explore various factors, individual, interpersonal, and structural that impact HIV-testing behaviors among AAPI, we utilized a social ecological framework to provide the theoretical foundation for this study. Ecological Systems Theory "asserts that human development is a product of interaction between the growing human organism and its environment" (Bronfenbrenner, 1979, p. 16). The theory suggests that individual development is impacted by micro, mezzo, and macro level systems within their environment. Micro level constitutes of systems that have the most immediate and direct impact on an individual; mezzo level constitutes systems that are of intermediate scale, and macro level includes entire communities and social systems. In the case of correlates of HIV testing in the AAPI community, microsystem factors would include perceived susceptibility, HIV knowledge, internalized HIV/AIDS stigma, etc.; mezzo level factors would include family, peer/social networks etc.; and, macrosystem factors would include institutionalized HIV/AIDS stigma, AAPI culture, etc. This theory allows us to identify factors at the different levels and to explore the interplay between them. The following review of literature is organized by the various micro-, mezzo-, and macro- level factors that impact HIV testing among AAPI. Since there is a lacuna of research on HIV among AAPI, we have included research from early 2000s. We also noticed that some authors treat AAPI as a monolithic group, while others focus on specific subgroups such as South East Asians, Asian Indians, Chinese, and also distinguish between American-or foreign–born. We include all of these studies in our review and indicate when authors or research identify results based on a specific subgroup of the AAPI community.

Individual or Micro-Factors

As in any other population groups, HIV knowledge and perception of HIV risk are two main factors that impact HIV testing in the AAPI population. However, it is noteworthy that, overall, AAPI demonstrate a low level of knowledge and high levels of misconception about HIV transmission. It should also be noted that studies on HIV knowledge and perception in this community have tended to focus on youth.

As early as 2000, Bhattacharya, Cleland and Holland's study on American-born Asian Indian adolescents found that while 86% of the participants knew that unsafe sexual practices with an HIV positive individual could transmit HIV, 47% did not know that sharing a razor could do the same, and 27% and 14% believed that donating blood and taking blood tests could transmit HIV respectively. In fact, the participant's level of HIV transmission knowledge was limited to modes of transmission such as unprotected anal and vaginal intercourse. The participants reported a low level of knowledge regarding other modes of transmission such as oral sex and breastfeeding. The authors also noted that some participants believed that only gay men can contract HIV and that marriage can prevent it. Similar trends were identified by a study on HIV testing behaviors among a sample of 604 Southeast Asians living in an urban setting in the U.S. and greater knowledge about HIV was associated with being more likely to have ever been tested for HIV (Huang et al., 2008).

Wong, and DeLeon's (2005) study on Asian American college students found that while participants reported low events of high-risk sexual behaviors, they also reported a low level of knowledge and concern about HIV/AIDS. The study participants demonstrated a low level of basic information regarding HIV transmission, risk, and prevention. Data indicated that the lifetime prevalence of unprotected sex was 37%. Data also indicated that lifetime drug use was associated with 30-day and lifetime Sexual Risk indices.

Acculturation has been identified as one of the factors that impact open conversations about sexually risky behaviors, thus, in turn, impacting HIV-related knowledge. Chung et al. (2007) found that more acculturated families have greater parent–child communication about sexually risky behavior. Conversely, researchers have found that less acculturated Chinese–American parents believe that talking about sex with children encourages early sexual activities, thereby avoiding any conversation around safe sex practices (Lee, Salman, & Wang, 2012). A study of health beliefs, sexual behaviors, and HIV risk among acculturated Taiwanese immigrants suggested that self-efficacy was the strongest predictor of sexual behavior and acculturation moderated health seeking behavior (Lin, Simoni, & Zemon, 2005).

Gender is another factor impacting HIV knowledge and testing in AAPI communities. A study on South East Asian women indicated that although these women may have high levels of HIV knowledge, their ability to navigate safe sex behaviors and HIV testing might be limited. Traditional sexual norms in this community prevent women from engaging in discussions about condom use, which in turn may prevent discussion about sexual health and knowledge. Moreover, married women might mistakenly assume that they were protected against HIV because they assumed that marriage equated monogamy (Bhattacharya, 2004; Gagnon, Merry, Bocking, Rosenberg, & Oxman-Martinez, 2010). Interestingly, AAPI women were more concerned about premarital pregnancy than HIV and were more prone to use contraceptive pills rather than to use condoms (DiStefano et al., 2012).

Yet another individual level factor impacting testing in the AAPI population along with low levels of knowledge and misconception about HIV transmission is a low perception of HIV-risk. AAPI often perceive that they are at low levels of risk for HIV infection (Yoshikawa et al., 2003). One of the main misconceptions in the AAPI community is that HIV/AIDS does not impact heterosexual populations (Bhattacharya, Cleland, & Holland, 2000). DiStefano et al., (2012) reported that in AAPI communities, heterosexuality is often equated to monogamy and thus deemed free from HIV-related risk. Finally, within many Asian communities, HIV is viewed as a "White disease" (Yoshikawa et al., 2003) or an "illness of foreigners" (Kang, Rapkin, Springer, & Kim, 2003). This may further help to explain the low level of perceived susceptibility within the AAPI communities.

Mezzo Level Factors

The key player in this dimension is social support, which includes family and peer relations. In a collectivist culture such as AAPI, family norms and traditions are an integral part of one's self-concept. Every individual occupies a certain position within the family system and is responsible for fulfilling family obligations that include enhancing a family's reputation in the community (Bhattacharya, 2004). This also means that individual behavior reflects on the family and community. Within this context, even seeking health care for HIV/AIDS can be seen as bringing shame on family and community. In the AAPI culture, HIV/AIDS represents a deviation from the cultural norms and mores in several ways. It is closely connected to aberrant sexual behaviors such as multiple sexual partners or homosexuality; both considered taboo in Asian cultures, where traditional sexual norms are linked to procreation and maintaining family lineage (Yoshika & Schustak, 2001). In addition, sex is considered a private matter and thus not something to be discussed in either familial or community settings (Chng et al., 2003). Therefore, a sexually transmitted infection such as HIV/AIDS is connected to issues of privacy, vulnerability, and possible identification with a stigmatized role. It also represents the fear of disrupting family relationships, of being a burden (if found HIV positive), as well as fear of discrimination within the family and community (Wilson & Yoshikawa, 2004). This is particularly true for AAPI MSM because for them acknowledging HIV risk would also likely mean acknowledging homosexuality to their families (Do, Hudes, Proctor, Han, & Choi, 2006). Thus, the potential shame and loss of face become important motivators for not seeking HIV testing (Vlassoff & Ali, 2011). It is therefore not surprising that research indicates that HIV disclosure experiences by AAPI are influenced by emotional self-protection and desire to conceal one's own sexual orientation. Thus, many individuals choose not to disclose to family members because of stigma, a lack of HIV-related awareness of family members and avoidance of unpleasant interaction (Kang, Rapkin, & DeAlmeida, 2006). On the other hand, individuals often choose to inform their friends because peers represent a source of positive support. Thus, in the absence of family support, friendship networks become one of the few contexts in which AAPI may seek HIV-specific support or support in general (Yoshioka & Schustack, 2001).

Macro/Structural Factors

These factors include HIV-related stigma, provider discrimination and access to culturally grounded HIV-related services. The research on the mezzo-level factors indicated that cultural and sexual mores contribute to AAPI having a difficult time expressing their sexual behavior and sexuality within their communities. In fact, since heteronormity is considered the undisputed hegemony in the AAPI culture, the stigmatizing discourse around HIV/AIDS "allows members of the community to distance themselves and their self-defined in-groups from the risk of infection by blaming contraction of the illness on characteristics normally associated with out-group, who are classified as deviant or 'other'" (Deacon, 2006, p. 420). Thus, HIV/AIDS is constructed as preventable, immoral behaviors such as "promiscuity," "homosexuality" and "drug use" are identified as causing the illness, and such behaviors are associated with "carriers" who are to be blamed for their own infection which leads to potential status loss and discrimination of AAPI individuals seeking to HIV-related services including testing (Chin, Leung, Sheth, & Rodriguez, 2007; Kang, Rapkin, & DeAlmeida, 2006; Vlassoff & Ali, 2011).

Thus, in many cases, AAPI living with HIV/AIDS delay accessing medical and supportive services, report difficulties adhering to their antiretroviral regimen, experience psychological distress related to HIV stigma, and avoid disclosing their HIV status in fear of being discriminated against by peers, employers, and family members (Choi, Hann, Hudes, & Kegeles, 2002; Do et al., 2006; Lee, Ayers, & Kronenfeld, 2009; Stein & Nyamathi, 2000).

Another structural factor that few studies have addressed and could be an important determinant of HIV testing among AAPI is the availability of culturally sensitive and linguistically appropriate testing. However limited, research in this area indicates that knowing a comfortable place to undergo testing is significantly and positively associated with recent HIV testing (Do et al., 2006). This finding suggest that having information on culturally appropriate sources of care and testing facilities may influence the HIV-testing behaviors of AAPI.

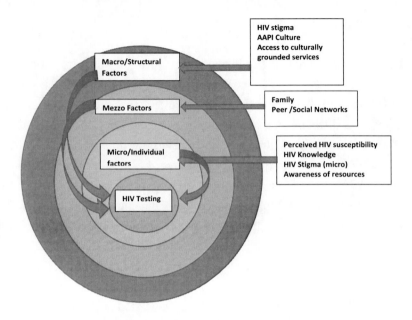

Figure 1. Thematic representation of the relational model between HIV testing behavior and micro, mezzo and macro factors.

Research on service provision suggests that the high proportion of immigrants in the AAPI population presents challenges for HIV service providers, particularly in ensuring that current services can adequately meet the needs of diverse AAPI subgroups. Because of varying histories of migrations to the U.S. and reasons for immigration (e.g., seeking employment or seeking political refuge), AAPI ethnic groups have different levels of language proficiencies, levels of wealth, and health coverage (Chin, Kang, Kim, Martinez, & Eckholdt, 2006). Furthermore, AAPI experience both subtle and overt discrimination on the basis of race, immigration status, and sexual orientation. In a recent study comparing non-Hispanic Whites and other racial/ethnic minorities, including AAPI, in terms of perceived provider discrimination, results indicate that the latter group report more perceived provider discrimination (Lee et al., 2009) and because of this perception this group is more likely to delay health seeking, resulting in poorer health outcomes in general and HIV/AIDS-related outcomes in particular. Figure 1 provides a thematic representation of the various factors and their impact on HIV testing.

METHODS

This mixed-methods study utilized both quantitative and qualitative methods to meet two aims: 1) to describe and 2) to examine in depth the correlates impacting testing behavior among AAPIs. To address the first aim, self-administered surveys were used to collect data from 75 participants on demographics and the various correlates of HIV testing (that were identified through the literature review including HIV knowledge, HIV risk, and HIV-related stigma). To address the second aim, narrative data were collected from a subsample of 10 randomly selected participants to obtain a more in-depth information on these factors.

Procedures

The institutional review board at San Jose State University reviewed and approved study procedures. Participants were community members that met all of the following inclusion criteria for entry into the study: 1) self-identification as AAPI, 2) at least 18 years old, 3) engage in risk behaviors, and, 4) able to speak and understand English. This project was done in collaboration with a community-based organization in the Bay Area that has been providing HIV-related services to AAPI population for forty years. Our community partner was responsible for screening and recruitment of participants. Since this was a hard to reach population, sampling methods used were convenience and snowball. Participants were recruited through a variety of methods, such as community outreach (e.g., health fairs, bathhouses, community organizations, community boards, local "hang out" spots, clinics/social services, and other locations) as well as through social networking sites. Potential participants provided verbal consent to participate in a brief screening to determine study eligibility at venues or by telephone. Upon meeting the inclusion criteria, appointments for the quantitative data collection were made.

We used a systematic random sampling method to arrive at our subsample for the qualitative arm. Since we were aiming to collect data from 10 individuals, we selected 7 as the random number for selecting participants for the qualitative arm. Thus the 7th, 14th, 21st participants and so on were selected to partake in the interviews until we reached the sample size 10. Written consent from all participants was obtained before data collection for both the quantitative and qualitative study arms.

Data Collection and Instruments

Quantitative data were collected through self-administered surveys. Qualitative interviews were conducted using a semistructured questionnaire by the Principle Investigators and trained research assistants. For the self-administered surveys, research assistants were available to answer any questions. Interviews were digitally recorded and transcribed. Participants were given $10 for completing the surveys and an additional $20 gift card for participating in the face-to-face interview. The survey instruments and the domains of the semistructured interview schedule were guided by the literature review. The following validated instruments that have been used extensively among AAPI were utilized for this study: (a) Screening Form: A screening form containing the study inclusion and exclusion criteria was administered to potential eligible individuals, (b) Demographic Questionnaire, (c) Risk Behavior Survey, (d) HIV Testing History, (e) HIV-Knowledge Questionnaire, and (f) HIV Stigma Questionnaire. Each of these questionnaires had multiple questions on them. The risk behavior questionnaire asked about number of partners (casual or regular), condom use, and intravenous drug use. The testing behavior questionnaire asked if the participant has been tested in the past year and what were the barriers and facilitators to testing. The HIV-knowledge questionnaire had questions on transmission and prevention. The HIV-Stigma questionnaire had questions based on personalized attitudes and public attitudes toward people with HIV including fear of contagion and stigmatizing views of individuals with HIV. These questionnaires were guided by research and modified from the questionnaires developed by the CDC and the Population Council, thus, ensuring reliability and validity of the instruments.

Informed by the review of literature, the semi-structured interview guide included both individual and contextual factors that may influence HIV-testing behaviors, such as fear of disclosure, stigmatization, perception of susceptibility, language needs, role of family, religious beliefs, cultural norms, social networks, and community services.

Data Analysis

A code book for the quantitative data was developed and data were entered into SPSS. Descriptive analyses were performed to describe participant background characteristics and responses to the various survey instruments.

To analyze qualitative data, we utilized the grounded theory approach developed by Glasser and Strauss (1967). This inductive method has four components: (a) data collection and analysis occur concurrently, (b) collected data are coded according to themes that emerge from the data, (c) theoretical and methodological memos are written and become part of the data to analyze, and, (d) codes are conceptually linked to generate explanatory frameworks. This inductive approach is used to generate theory from data, rather than to test existing hypotheses.

The first step in the coding process involved open coding and discussion of the emerging themes. Using a content analysis approach, readers refined their notions about the themes and potential ways of coding the responses. Thematic codes were developed inductively as successive transcripts were reviewed, allowing the data to dictate the analytic categories. Readers continued reading and revising until no new codes emerged from the data. Through this iterative process of coding, review, discussion, and revision, thematic codes were documented in a code book for categorizing responses. Research staff took several steps to increase methodological rigor: (a) multiple researchers participated in data coding and analysis to ensure multiple viewpoints and discussion of perceptions of data, (b) evaluators sought consensus on coder agreement to ensure more accurate coding. Once all of the transcripts were coded, passages coded with individual themes were extracted from the dataset for analysis.

RESULTS

Sample

This mixed-methods study included 75 AAPI who completed the questionnaires and a subset of 10 individuals who were randomly selected for the qualitative arm of the study. The sample consisted of 89% Asian Americans and 11% Pacific Islanders. Almost 60% were male, 90% were between 18 and 34 years old, 63% were U.S. born, 55% spoke English at home (followed by 32% who spoke Vietnamese), 57% never married or were single, 41% had a 4-year college degree and 31% had some college education, 60% were employed, 50% lived with families and friends, 32% identified as Catholic), followed by 15% Buddhist, 14% had no religious affiliations, and 18% abstained from answering this question). Table 1 in the appendix provides a more detailed breakdown of the demographic data.

Descriptive Statistics

Frequencies were run on the various survey variables to see how these variables were distributed and to address the first research questions. Each of the surveys had multiple questions. Here, we present descriptive statistics on the most relevant findings. With regard to risk behaviors, it is interesting to note that although all participants screened for this study qualified based on engagement in HIV-risk behavior within the past year, 71% ($n = 39$) reported that they had engaged in risky behavior that might expose them to HIV/AIDS within the past year and the remaining 29% ($n = 16$) believed that they had not engaged in any HIV-related risk behavior over the past year. On an average, the participants reported having sex with more than four individuals, having utilized condoms twice with a regular partner and three times with casual partners over the past 30 days.

Interestingly, only 55% ($n = 41$) of the participants reported having received HIV testing in the past year. On the checklist of potential barriers to HIV testing, endorsement of barriers ranged from 19% to 90%.

Table 1. Demographic Characteristics of Participants (N = 75)

Demographic variables	% (N)
Gender	
Male	58.7 (44)
Female	40.0 (30)
Transgender	1.3 (1)
Age	
18 – 24	53.3 (40)
25 – 34	37.4 (28)
35 – 44	5.3 (4)
45 – 54	4.0 (3)
Race/Ethnicity	
Asian	89.3 (67)
Native Hawaiian/Pacific Islander	10.7 (8)
Country of Origin	
USA	63.5 (47)
Vietnam	21.6 (16)
Philippines	5.3 (4)
Cambodia	1.4 (1)
China	1.4 (1)
Hong Kong	1.4 (1)
Japan	1.4 (1)
Laos	1.4 (1)
South Korea	1.4 (1)
Taiwan	1.4 (1)
Years Lived in USA	
<1	1.4 (1)
1-5	4.0 (3)
5-10	2.7 (2)
11-20	35.1 (26)
21-30	48.7 (36)
31-40	6.7 (5)
41-50	1.4 (1)
Language Spoken at Home	
English	55.4 (41)
Cantonese	1.4 (1)
Language Spoken at Home	% N
Chinese	5.4 (4)
Mandarin	1.4 (1)
Vietnamese	32.4 (24)
Samoan	1.4 (1)
Tagalog	1.4 (1)
Sexual Orientation	
Homosexual	21.3 (16)
Bisexual	13.4 (10)
Gay, Lesbian, Queer or Same Gender Loving	8.0 (6)

Demographic variables	% (N)
Straight/Heterosexual	56.0 (42)
I do not know my sexual orientation	1.3 (1)
Marital Status	
Never Married	92.0 (69)
Separated	4.0 (3)
A member of an unmarried couple	2.7 (2)
Divorced	1.3 (1)
Education	
Grade 12 or GED (High school graduate)	16.4 (12)
College 1-3 years (Some college or technical school)	38.4 (28)
College 4 years (College graduate)	41.1 (30)
Graduate School (Advanced degree)	4.1 (3)
Employment Status	
Employed for wages	60.8 (45)
Self-employed	4.1 (3)
Out of work	6.7 (5)
A homemaker	1.4 (1)
A student	27.0 (20)
Hoursehold income	
Less than $10,000	25.4 (18)
$10,000 to $19,999	16.9 (12)
$20,000 to $29,999	11.2 (8)
$30,000 to $39,999	16.9 (12)
$40,000 to $49,999	4.2 (3)
$50,000 to $69,999	12.7 (9)
$70,000 to $89,999	4.2 (3)
$100,000 to $149,000	7.1 (5)
Current Living Situation	
Homeless	1.3 (1)
Staying with relatives/friends	50.7 (38)
Renting	36.0 (27)
Own home	12.0 (9)
Religious Background	
Christian	8.3 (6)
Atheist	6.9 (5)
Catholic	31.9 (23)
Agnostic	4.2 (3)
Buddhist	15.3 (11)
Seventh Day Adventist	1.4 (1)
None	13.9 (10)
Prefer not to answer	18.1 (13)

The most frequently endorsed barriers to testing were the perception of an HIV-negative status (90%, $n = 63$), a belief that one has not had a drug-related risk behavior that would expose one to HIV (84%, $n = 59$), a perception of low or no HIV risk (83%, $n = 59$) and the belief that one had not had a sexually risky encounter that would cause HIV exposure (80%, $n = 56$). Other endorsed barriers included denial of thinking about the possibility of a positive status (67%, $n = 46$), fear of upsetting family members (61%, $n = 43$), fear of who might find out about their HIV status (60%, $n = 42$) and a fear of finding out one's HIV positive status (58%, $n = 40$) as well as not wanting others to think that the individual was a drug user (40%, $n = 20$). The items that had a lower endorsement rate included not having time to get tested (25%, $n = 17$), not having anyone to talk to about getting tested (23%, $n = 16$), and not knowing where to get tested (20%, $n = 14$). Of the 34 (45%) who got tested, 15% gave the reason for getting tested as wanting to know their status, 12% cited unsafe sex as the reason, 10% wanted to protect oneself or be safe, and 8% received testing as part of a general health checkup or physical. A majority of the 34 respondents (80%) were tested on their own volition, whereas 12% were encouraged by friends and 8% by a medical service provider. Sixty percent of participants described their experience of getting tested as easy, good, pleasant, or convenient; 18% were neutral; 5% reported a mixed experience (e.g., nervous but good, or good but scary); and 17% indicated that their experience was embarrassing, intimidating, scary, or devastating.

A 45-item HIV-knowledge questionnaire was used to collect data on this variable. The responses to the questions on the scale were recoded as correct and incorrect. Almost 25% ($n = 19$) of the study's participants responded incorrectly on 29 of the 45 items on the questionnaire. The items with the most incorrect answers were "HIV is killed by bleach" (85%, $n = 63$), "Women are always tested for HIV during their pap smears" (71%, $n = 53$), and "HIV can be spread by mosquitoes" (68%, $n = 51$). The questions where participants demonstrated the most knowledge and provided a correct answer were "Using a latex condom or rubber can lower a person's chance of getting HIV" (92%, $n = 69$), "You can usually tell if someone has HIV by looking at them" (92%, $n = 69$), "A woman can get HIV if she has vaginal sex with a man who has HIV" (92%, $n = 69$), and "Having sex with more than one partner can increase a person's chance of being infected with HIV" (91%, $n = 68$).

In terms of HIV stigma, 19% ($n = 14$) of participants reported having a lot of fear and 40% ($n = 30$) reported having a little fear, while the remaining 41% ($n = 31$) reported having no fear of becoming infected with HIV from sharing a drinking glass with a person with HIV. Twenty-nine percent ($n = 22$) indicated that they would not buy fresh vegetables from a shopkeeper or vendor they knew had HIV, and 55% ($n = 41$) indicated that they would rather not touch someone with HIV because they are scared of infection. A majority of the participants (64%, $n = 48$) believed that people with HIV are promiscuous and almost half of the participants (48%, $n = 36$) asserted that injection drug users should be blamed for spreading HIV. Thirty-three percent ($n = 25$) believed that AIDS was a punishment for bad behavior, 41% ($n = 31$) were of the view that a person with AIDS must have done something wrong, 33% ($n = 25$) blamed female sex workers for spreading HIV, 31% ($n = 23$) reported that individuals who contract HIV through high-risk behaviors deserve what they get. Twenty-nine percent ($n = 22$) reported that women get HIV because they are prostitutes and 21% ($n = 16$) understood homosexuality to be the cause of HIV.

Qualitative Themes

Five focal issues could be gleaned from the ten randomly chosen participants' narratives: generational difference and parental expectations regarding sexuality, HIV knowledge gained outside the family environment, facilitators to HIV testing, barriers to HIV testing, and HIV education as a recommendation.

Generational Difference and Parental Expectations Regarding Sexuality

Most participants recognized that their own more acculturated values regarding sexuality and sexual behaviors were in conflict with the traditional values of their parents' generations. In their opinions, these traditional values created assumptions among parents regarding their children's sexual orientation and monogamy. These assumptions, in turn, led to parents having expectations that the children would abstain from sexually risky behavior, would get married, and have a family. Some of these tensions are reflected in the comments below:

> "...I'm okay being on my own, and that's why I don't have to feel like you have to be with a partner or get married. Which I think is bad because...'cause ultimately that's what we're supposed to be here for...to get married and have kids but I really don't think that way."

> "I hope they don't think of me that their son is sexually active. I think that's just their mentality. They would not rather—"oh he's a hard worker, he works at this company" not just "oh, is my son having protected sex?"

Participants also shared the notion that their parents' generation was more monogamous and therefore any discussions regarding HIV knowledge and risks with them seemed moot.

> "They're (my parents) of a different generation, as far as I know, they have only had one sexual partner for the past 30 years. So, I mean, probably, it (HIV) isn't a concern to them. So, it's not something that they need to know...I don't think they would even care."

According to the participants, this perceived monogamous nature of the older generation also impacted the discussion of HIV testing and HIV-prevention strategies. In fact, two of the 10 participants indicated that any HIV or sexually transmitted infection (STI) prevention programs in their communities only target the younger generations.

> "... my parents are married and they are happy together. So if you were to ask them to go get tested, they're not going to be like, "I'm with my husband, I'm with my wife. Why would I need to do that?" They don't understand that people sleep around and that you know, they cheat, and they're still like that.

> I mean if you see an ad about AIDS or whatever, 'have you gotten tested?' It's always a younger male younger female, early 20s maybe early 30s. It's never a person around our parents' age. It's not something towards their focus. I guess you could say."

These cultural norms and expectations made any conversations regarding sex, drugs, and HIV with parents almost prohibitive. All participants talked about coming from a culture that does not condone any open discussion of topics on substance use, mental health, sex, and HIV. They acknowledged that the Western cultural norms of having open discussions between parents and children regarding sexuality and sexual health were not common in AAPI communities. All alluded to the taboo surrounding such topics and their unpleasant nature. In fact, they were of the view that such discussions may even lead to their parents assuming that their children may be engaging in behaviors that were not culturally congruent.

> "I think it's kind of our culture to just not talk about things like that. Like I have never heard of an Asian family talking about sex before at least to their kids…at least the first generation Asian family and I also never heard a family talk about drugs either so it's just kind of taboo in our culture."

This idea of "culture of silence" around topics of sexuality and risky behaviors led to the next theme that emerged from the interviews.

HIV Knowledge Is Gained Outside the Family Environment

While all participants were knowledgeable about HIV and its transmission routes, they unanimously mentioned having received this information outside the family context through their peers, media, and at school. They reported that their first formal discussion regarding topics on sexuality typically occurred within their school settings and with peers of the same age and similar identities.

"... sex classes, my peers. A lot from my peers didn't really talk about it in their family 'cause we didn't talk about those things. Yeah, mostly from my peers and school."

"Sex education has brought some information there. I was also part of Queer and Asian Club at a College in CA and we had meetings about HIV and we did bring some stuff up about that (sex). I learned some stuff from class—from human sexuality as well."

Interestingly, most of the participants also identified the internet, TV shows, and social media as other popular avenues of gathering HIV-related knowledge. Following are some illustrative comments:

"The television show Queer as Folk—it brought in the subject of HIV and they did talk about the medicines that they have to help manage HIV and viral loads. That was my first exposure to the drugs and then I did do some research myself on it…"

"Magic Johnson … Everyone knows, or at least when like you watch basketball you'd know."

Despite the fact that there was a common recognition of taboo around the topics of sexuality and HIV, all 10 participants reported having been tested twice for HIV throughout their lifetime. They were all aware of where to get tested and alluded to a general satisfaction with regard to the overall testing experience. We present here two themes that emerged from the discussion on HIV testing; *factors that facilitate testing* and *factors that act as barriers to testing*. Despite describing their testing experience as quick and easy, participants also spoke of feelings of fear and anxiety as they waited for their test result.

Facilitators to HIV Testing

The most common reason cited by the participants for wanting to get tested was their partners' risky behaviors. These risk factors, according to the respondents, included "being bisexual," "being promiscuous," and "using drugs." The following comments reflect this viewpoint:

> "I was seeing a guy then I realized that he was bisexual and was seeing other people as well. So and he was using drugs, different drugs that I wasn't using. So I really want to just be sure that I didn't catch anything."

> "I wanted a relationship, and he just took advantage of me. And then found that he's a promiscuous person and that he likes to sleep around. So that made me really nervous."

Wanting to know their HIV status and motivation to maintain HIV negative status also played important roles in their decision to get tested. It appeared that their knowledge of HIV has been a positive contributor to their testing decisions.

> "Condoms are not 100% proof for HIV and then, you know, I mean, I knew I was negative, but you know, there's nothing, there's that small percentage I could be infected and it's better to be safe than sorry."

> "It was just 'cause I have never been tested my whole life. Worried about my status and then after that, it was just trying to maintain my status in a way and I want to know it every so often."

Barriers to HIV Testing

Although all participants unanimously mentioned HIV-related stigma as the greatest barrier to getting tested, they themselves did not ascribe to the attitudes. The respondents spoke of various levels of stigma; individual, familial, and cultural. This stigma often gave rise to fear of finding out their status because a positive status could mean loss of social networks and social support, particularly in the context of cultural and familial norms that inhibited open conversations around safe sex and sexual matters. Thus, the potential shame and loss of face may become important motivators for not seeking HIV testing, as is illustrated by the following comments:

"… they're scared of the outcome. They're afraid that someone is going to find out and may think badly of them."

"Fear. I think one of the big things is fear like they don't want to know that they're positive or not…sometimes it's too hard."

The participants also shared the view that within the broader AAPI culture, HIV was intricately linked to "promiscuity" and this put the onus of contracting HIV solely on individual behavior. Such attitudes were reflected in phrases such as "you did it to yourself" or "you are sleeping around."

"… because if you need to get tested you're probably being reckless. That's why my mom would say."

"Stigma that whoever has it is probably like, irresponsible, or very promiscuous. Just wasn't thinking. That's what they (family members) would think. I mean for me, I know you can contract it many different ways…"

From such stigmatizing views arose shame of being perceived as someone engaging in risky behavior.

"Maybe they just feel shameful. But it depends on their situation. Like, do they sleep around? Do they do drugs? Do they shoot needles? Do they do something that they're just ashamed if they're embarrassed about? They don't want to get tested."

"… they don't want their status to be out in the open to people and then you have to be in the waiting room with other people waiting for their results or waiting for their tests. It's sort of awkward. It's like saying, "Hey, look, I have unprotected sex or I've done something that put me in danger."

Participants who identified as part of LGBTQ communities acknowledged that these ideas of stigma and shame were rendered more complex within the context of these communities as a result of the intersectionality of multiple minority identities, racial/ethnic and sexual. These experiences became even more harmful when religion that condemned same-sex partnerships entered the equation.

> "… they (my family) probably think it's, I guess it just feeds to all of the gay promiscuity stereotypes and that all gays are promiscuous; and if they are they can contract this (HIV). That's probably what my parents think."
>
> "My friends think it's a gay thing, but these are friends that don't really accept a gay culture in a way… probably that one of them (stigma) is if you have a lot of sex like you are more of a whore than others, but then that's not necessarily true because you can get HIV with just one encounter…"
>
> "I'm Catholic… it's like people just look down on people who have like the sense of that like, "Hey you get this that means that you know you're promiscuous." 'Cause that's what they (religious individuals) think."
>
> "… I think too for Christian people, they think that if they are okay with it (concepts of HIV), they are supporting unsafe sex. I guess that could be a stigma there, sort of like promoting unsafe sex if you're okay with HIV."

Interestingly, another major barrier identified through the interviews was in the area of provider level stigma. There was a general consensus that many of the primary care providers were ill equipped to have conversations around sexuality and HIV-risk with their clients. This was particularly true if the primary care physician was also an AAPI individual.

> "… everywhere you go, you can still see providers that do not want to serve this population. Or they refer them immediately, because, they… well first they are not specialized for HIV care. But you can tell that they just want to move it over to infectious disease. There's still a lot of stigma out there."

"... So with primary care providers, I think there is a lot of times where people don't feel the most comfortable to ask about HIV because that could be linked to them revealing their sexuality and there is still a lot of stigma I think around sexuality."

HIV-Related Education and Awareness as a Recommendation

All participants identified the potential benefits of HIV-related education and awareness to reducing stigma and increasing testing among AAPI. They acknowledged that individual feelings of fear and shame that discourage HIV testing can be due to one's limited awareness of HIV and other sexually transmitted infections (STIs). They also associated their parents' "closed-mindedness" of HIV to low levels of education and awareness. Suggestions revolved around increasing knowledge and awareness as well as better integrating HIV and sexual health into primary care services.

"So moving more towards technology based or more online things might be more feasible applicable for the younger generation who are on their smart phone all the time and through other applications like Facebook, Twitter, Instagram, Snapchat, and so on."

"But I think being on the media, being on the air, is another way to engage because I think that a lot of time the older generation listen to radio. So maybe having that outlet, the media outlet, using the radio, using television or other communication channels that reach out to these generations."

In these responses, we see participants suggesting different avenues for educating different generations. They suggest an online and app-based approach for educating and engaging younger generations and TV and radio to connecting with the older generation. Additionally, members spoke about the need to integrate HIV as well as comprehensive sexual health services into the primary care setting.

"And so really if you are to look at it there needs to be more integration of this kind of work within the primary care providers and that they are seen at the same level."

DISCUSSION

This mixed-methods study identified and described various individual or micro, familial, peer relations or mezzo and cultural or macro factors that impact HIV-testing behaviors among AAPI. One of the inclusion criteria for the study was to screen for individuals with HIV-related risk behavior. Despite the fact that all 75 participants met this inclusion criterion, it is interesting to note that almost one-third of the sample did not believe that they had engaged in any risky behaviors in the past year. In addition, only half of the sample reported having received HIV testing in the past year. Our sample consisted of young, college educated AAPI individuals, very similar to the participants of the So, Wong, and DeLeon's (2005) study on Asian American college students. This study had found that while participants reported low events of high-risk sexual behaviors, they also reported a low level of knowledge and concern about HIV/AIDS. Interestingly, the results of our study conducted almost a decade later are still reflective of previous research indicating that AAPI often perceive themselves as having low risk for HIV infection (DeLeon, 2005; Yoshikawa et al., 2003). In fact, one of the most cited potential barriers to HIV testing (endorsed by 90% of the sample) was the perception that they are HIV-negative. This is not surprising given that lower levels of HIV-risk perception and testing are related to lower HIV knowledge (Di Stefano et al., 2012; Huang et al., 2008) and according to the results of this study, one-fifth of the sample answered more than 60% of the questions on the HIV knowledge questionnaire incorrectly.

Other major barriers to HIV testing that were identified were related to the fear of finding out one's positive status. Sixty-one percent of the sample were fearful of upsetting family members. This fear of disclosure is intricately linked to HIV-related stigma at the individual, familial, and cultural levels. These results are congruent with research that identify psychological distress related to HIV stigma and the fear of disclosing HIV status (Choi et al., 2002; Do et al., 2006; Lee et al., 2009; Yoshioka & Schustack, 2001). Stigmatizing perceptions toward HIV was reflected through the results, which indicated that 64% of the participants believed that people with HIV are promiscuous and almost half of the sample asserted that injection drug users should be blamed for the spread of HIV.

These quantitative results were corroborated by the qualitative findings as well. Through the qualitative in-depth interviews, we were able to obtain a glimpse of the culture-specific barriers to HIV testing, including cultural taboos against openly discussing sexual matters, and the association of HIV with homosexuality and nonmarital sex. Respondents shared the view that within the AAPI communities, individual behavior reflects on the larger family and/or community. In addition, highly personal and emotional topics are to be avoided because of their potential to cause embarrassment and discomfort. In their opinion, any discussion on sexual behavior and HIV would imply implicit disclosure of the fact that they may be engaging in risky behavior and thus bring disgrace and shame to their families. This led to a "culture of silence" around such topics. These results were reflected in studies focusing on cultural norms and traditions that might fuel HIV-related stigma in the AAPI communities (Chin, Leung, Sheth, & Rodriguez, 2007; Kang, Rapkin, & DeAlmeida, 2006; Vlassoff & Ali, 2011).

Tied to the idea of shaming the family was also the fear of losing family support. Family is a critical source of support in accordance with the importance of familial interdependence in many East Asian, Southeast Asian, and South Asian cultures (Bhattacharya, 2004; Chng et al., 2003; Kang, Rapkin, & DeAlmeida, 2006). Thus, according to the interview participants, many individuals may not choose to even discuss issues around sexuality and HIV, let alone disclose their sexual orientation or their HIV status to family members in order to protect them from the inherent shame and to avoid great personal loss.

There was a shared recognition that participants' own more acculturated views about sexuality are in conflict with the more traditional views of their parents, including monogamy, heterosexism, and premarital sex. Such views then created assumptions on the part of the parents that their children did not engage in premarital sex, would be monogamous and were heterosexual. Such assumptions coupled with a "culture of silence" around personal and emotional matters rendered any HIV-related discussion within the family almost redundant. Interestingly, the participants also viewed their parents' relationship as monogamous and long term, thereby perceiving low HIV risk in the parent generation. This was reflected in the research studies conducted by (Bhattacharya, 2004; Gagnon, Merry, Bocking, Rosenberg, & Oxman-Martinez, 2010). While prior literature has indicated the role of acculturation in HIV knowledge and testing, those studies were primarily focusing on the parent-child dyads and how high levels of acculturation led to more open conversations on sexuality and sexual health (Chung et. al. 2007; Lee, Salman, & Wang, 2012). Our study participants, however, spoke of a generational gap between parents and children moderated by acculturation.

The results of this study are indicative of certain research, policy, and practice implications that are outlined briefly in this section.

Research Implications

In order to change the help-seeking and testing behavior in this population, first is necessary to identify the sociocultural factors that impede such behavior. While this current study is an attempt in that direction, there is a significant paucity of data on these factors at the subgroup levels. Therefore, more pilot studies and other basic research on HIV-related subjects within the AAPI subethnic communities need to be conducted utilizing culturally relevant data collection methods. Studies that combine ethnography with quantitative methodologies might be better suited to help gather and analyze more culturally relevant data. For example, ethnographic data could elucidate information on specific cultural, familial, spiritual, psychosocial, and other contextual factors as they relate to the social and familial experiences of AAPI and their influence on AAPI' perceptions of HIV risk. These data could then be utilized to identify correlates to HIV-testing behavior and can be used to create larger, quantitative surveys.

The concept of stigma in and of itself is a complex one and is not well understood in the general population. However, it is even less understood in the AAPI community, where HIV-related stigma is compounded by other stigmatizing identities due to racism, homophobia, transphobia, etc. Much more research on stigmatized subgroups within AAPI communities such as intravenous drug users, MSM, and transgender individuals is necessary in order to understand the specific barriers to HIV testing and care faced by the most vulnerable at-risk AAPI. Given the exponential increase in new HIV diagnoses among AAPI MSM, future research targeting HIV stigma, risk behavior, and testing behavior among AAPI should be aimed at understanding the intersectional stigma and social discrimination experienced by AAPI MSM.

One of the greatest barriers to understanding stigma is its complex nature and a lack of common understanding of the concept across disciplines that are involved in the effort to combat stigma. Some researchers see it as a purely psychological process, while others come from a more sociological stance and see it as a society's way of reifying power structures (Parker & Aggleton, 2003). We would argue that in order to understand HIV related stigma in a more holistic manner, more research is needed that would combine both these micro and macro frameworks. Therefore, there is an urgent need for conceptual research that focuses on the concept of HIV stigma, specifically cultural manifestations of HIV stigma among AAPI. Conceptual research should also explore the applicability of layered or intersectional stigma models to the understanding of HIV stigma in these communities.

Policy Implications

This study found that participants reported not only general stigmatized views toward HIV-positive individuals, but also in regard to HIV and sex work, HIV and intravenous drug use, and HIV and nonheterosexual sex. This speaks to the need for structural level interventions in order to adequately target HIV-related stigma among AAPI. The study participants in the qualitative arm identified service-provider level stigma as a deterrent to HIV testing and recommended more stigma-reducing interventions including increase in knowledge and awareness in the community. They also recommended different venues for reaching different age groups. These recommendations can be utilized to modify current policies driving the HIV-related prevention and care. Advocacy is needed on national, state, and local policy levels in order to ensure support for activities focused on HIV-stigma-reduction campaigns tailored to AAPI. Social workers advocating for the needs of AAPI on a broad policy level, community systems level, and within individual community-based organizations should be aware of the specific vulnerabilities of HIV-positive and at-risk community members. Therefore, it is crucial that social service providers gain familiarity with current and proposed laws (such as health care and immigration reforms) as well as shifts in funding related to HIV.

Practice Implications

This study's findings indicate the need for culturally relevant HIV prevention and education among AAPI. The low rate of HIV testing (55%) compared with the reported level of risk behavior (71%) of the study sample illustrates the ineffectiveness of current prevention and education campaigns to reach at-risk AAPI. The salience of family as indicated by the participant narratives clearly illustrates that professionals need to be sensitive to potential isolation and fears of family intolerance and rejection. While typically, family may be a great source of support, it might not be so in this case. Thus, while approaches to intervention that integrate filial support can be explored, service providers need to be aware that their own values of including family in life events may be in conflict with those of their clients.

We would argue that the ultimate goal of interventions is social change, and in this case to reduce the disease burden among AAPI. Starting with assessment, through intervention, and into evaluation, clinicians can engage clients in an organic or ethnographic-based process in which they collaborate with social workers in identifying the sociocultural features that underpin HIV risk behavior while paying special attention to stigma. Green (1997) highlights the importance of cultural salience in problem definition and intervention selection. He refers to this factor as "what may be salient for clients, their way of comprehending and working with a problem, the "commonness" of their common sense... As "knowers", their experience is rich in matters that I know little or nothing of, but about which I need greater familiarity so I can better meet their needs" (p. 166). Therefore, as social service providers engaged in cross-cultural service provision, it is imperative that we understand both micro- as well as macro-level factors that influence risk and testing behaviors among AAPI.

CONCLUSION

Several limitations of the study should be acknowledged. This study was exploratory and the small sample sizes from each AAPI subgroup (Figure 1) did not allow us to make comparisons between groups. While the percentage of Pacific Islander in the study was relatively small (11%), it was reflective of the overall PI population size in the San Francisco Bay Area; however, this study has limited generalizability. This study also faced the challenge of focusing on the stigmatized subject of HIV. This was probably a significant barrier to recruitment of the study sample, not only in terms of reaching an adequate sample size but also in terms of the subject matter's influence on who was willing to participate in the study. Thus AAPI who held more stigmatized views toward HIV may have automatically opted out of participating in the study, and therefore their views were not reflected. The average age of the sample was 25 years, thus rendering the results somewhat skewed. In addition, we relied on self-reported outcome measures on the various surveys used. Thus, responses from the participants might have been biased by social desirability and cultural constraints against revealing private behaviors, which was reflected in the numbers on the risk-behavior question.

Despite these limitations, this study adds to the growing body of knowledge that focuses on understanding the various correlates to HIV testing among AAPI. By utilizing an ecological framework, this study identifies the various individual- and structural-level factors that impact HIV-testing behavior and suggests some interventions at various levels. Finally, this study highlights the importance of exploring family involvement in the HIV-prevention process and suggests the need for more culturally tailored intervention models that keep stigma at the center of any public health initiatives.

REFERENCES

[1] Adih, W. K., Campsmith, M., Williams, C. L., Hardnett, F. P., & Hughes, D. (2011). Epidemiology of HIV among Asians and Pacific Islanders in the United States, 2001–2008. *Journal of International Association of Physicians in AIDS Care*. Retrieved from http://xa.yimg.com/kq/groups/23413065/949207740/name/Adih%2520epi%2520among%2520Asians-PI.pdf.

[2] Bronfenbrenner, U. (1979). *The ecology of human development*. Cambridge, MA: Harvard University Press.

[3] Bhattacharya, G. (2004). Health care seeking for HIV/AIDS among South Asians in the United States. *Health & Social Work, 29*(2), 106–115.

[4] Bhattacharya, G., Cleland, C., & Holland, S. (2000). Knowledge about HIV/AIDS, the perceived risks of infection and sources of information of Asian–Indian adolescents born in the USA. *AIDS Care, 12*(2), 203–209.

[5] Centers for Disease Control and Prevention. (2014). *Effective HIV surveillance among Asian Americans and Native Hawaiians and other Pacific Islanders*. Retrieved from http://www.cdc.gov/hiv/pdf/policies_13_238558_hivsurveillance_nhas_v6_508.pdf on 6/26/17.

[6] Centers for Disease Control and Prevention (2015). *HIV Surveillance Report vol. 27*. Retrieved from http://www.cdc.gov/hiv/library/reports/hiv-surveillance.html on 6/26/17.

[7] Centers for Disease Control and Prevention. (2016a). *HIV among Asians.* Retrieved from http://www.cdc.gov/hiv/group/racialethnic/asians/index.html on 6/1/17.

[8] Chin, J. J., Leung, M., Sheth, L., & Rodriguez, T. R. (2007). Let's not ignore a growing HIV problem for Asian and Pacific Islanders in the U.S. *Journal of Urban Health, 84*(5), 642–647. doi:10.1007/s11524-007-9200-8.

[9] Chng, C. L., Wong, F. Y., Park, R. J., Edberg, M. C., & Lai, D. S. (2003). A Model of Understanding Sexual Health among Asian American/Pacific Islander Men Who Have Sex With Men (MSM) in the United States. *AIDS Education and Prevention,* 15, Supplement A, 21-38.

[10] Choi, K. H., Hann, C. S., Hudes, E. S., & Kegeles, S. (2002). Unprotected sex and associated risk factors among young Asian and Pacific Islander men who have sex with men. *AIDS Education and Prevention, 14*(6), 472–481.

[11] Chung, P. J., Travis Jr., R., Kilpatrick, S. D., Elliott, M. N., Lui, C., Khandwala, S. B., & Schuster, M. A. (2007). Acculturation and parent–adolescent communication about sex in Filipino–American families: A community-based participatory research study. *Journal of Adolescent Health, 40*(6), 543–550.

[12] Deacon, H. (2006). Towards a sustainable theory of health-related stigmas: Lessons from the HIV/AIDS literature. *Journal of Community and Applied Social Psychology,* 16, 418-425.

[13] DiStefano, A. S., Hui, B., Barrera-Ng, A., Quitugua, L. F., Peters, R., Dimaculangan, J., Tanjasiri, S. P. (2012). Contextualization of HIV and HPV risk and prevention among Pacific Islander young adults in Southern California. *Social Science & Medicine, 75*(4), 699–708.

[14] Do, T. D., Hudes, E. S., Proctor, K., Han, C., & Choi, K. (2006). HIV testing and correlates among young Asian and Pacific Islander men who have sex with men in two U.S. cities. *AIDS Education and Prevention, 18*(1), 44–55.

[15] Gagnon, A. J., Merry, L., Bocking, J., Rosenberg, E., & Oxman-Martinez, J. (2010). South Asian migrant women and HIV/STIs:

knowledge, attitudes and practices and the role of sexual power. *Health & Place, 16*(1), 10–15.
[16] Glaser, B. and Strauss, A. L. (1967). *The Discovery of Grounded Theory: Strategies for*
[17] *Qualitative Research.* Chicago: Aldine De Gruyter.
[18] Green, J. W. (1998). *Cultural awareness in the human services: A multi-ethnic approach* (3rd ed.). Boston, MA: Allyn and Bacon.
[19] Huang, Z. J., Wong, F. Y., De Leon, J. M., & Park, R. J. (2008). Self-reported HIV testing behaviors among a sample of Southeast Asians in an urban setting in the United States. *AIDS Education and Prevention, 20*(1), 65–77.
[20] Kang, E., Rapkin, B. D., Springer, C., & Kim, J. H. (2003). The "demon plague" and access to care among Asian undocumented immigrants living with HIV disease in New York City. *Journal of Immigrant Health, 5*(2), 49–58.
[21] Kang, E., Rapkin, B. D., & DeAlmeida, C. (2006). Are psychological consequences of stigma enduring or transitory? A longitudinal study of HIV stigma and distress among Asians and Pacific Islanders living with HIV illness. *AIDS Patient Care & STDs, 20*(10), 712–723.
[22] Lee, Y., Salman, A., & Wang, F. (2012). Recruiting Chinese American adolescents to HIV/AIDS-related research: A lesson learned from a cross-sectional study. *Applied Nursing Research, 25*(1), 40-46.
[23] Lin, P., Simoni, J. M., & Zemon, V. (2005). The health belief model, sexual behaviors, and HIV risk among Taiwanese immigrants. *AIDS Education & Prevention, 17*(5), 469-483.
[24] Lee, C., Ayers, S. L., & Kronenfeld, J. J. (2009). The association between perceived provider discrimination, health care utilization and health status in racial and ethnic minorities. *Ethnicity & Disease, 19*(3), 330–337.
[25] Operario, D., & Nemoto, T. (2005). Sexual risk behavior and substance use among a sample of Asian Pacific Islander transgendered women. *AIDS Education & Prevention, 17*(5), 430-443.

[26] Parker, R., & Aggleton, P. (2003). HIV and AIDS-related stigma and discrimination: A conceptual framework and implications for action. *Social Science & Medicine, 57*(1), 13-24.

[27] So, D. W., Wong, F. Y., & DeLeon, D. M. (2005). Sex, HIV risks, and substance use among Asian American college students. *AIDS Education and Prevention, 17*(5), 457-468.

[28] Stein, J. A., & Nyamathi, A. (2000). Gender differences in behavioral and psychosocial predictors of HIV testing and return for test results in a high-risk population. *AIDS Care, 12*, 343–356.

[29] Trieu, S. L., Modeste, N. N., Marshak, H. H., Males, M. A., & Bratton, S. I. (2008). Factors associated with the decision to obtain an HIV test among Chinese/Chinese American community college women in Northern California. *Californian Journal of Health Promotion, 6*(1), 111–127.

[30] United States Census Bureau. (2013). *Asians fastest-growing race or ethnic group in 2012 [Press release]*. Retrieved from http://www.census.gov/newsroom/releases/archives/population /cb13-112.html.

[31] Vlassoff, C., & Ali, F. (2011). HIV-related stigma among South Asians in Toronto. *Ethnicity & Health, 16*(1), 25–42. doi:10.1080/13557858.2010.523456.

[32] Wilson, P. A., & Yoshikawa, H. (2004). Experiences of and responses to social discrimination among Asian and Pacific Islander gay men: Their relationship to HIV risk. *AIDS Education & Prevention, 16*(1), 68-83.

[33] Wong, F. Y., Campsmith, M. L., Nakamura, G. V., Crepaz, N., & Begley, E. (2004). HIV testing and awareness of care-related services among a group of HIV+ Asian Americans and Pacific Islanders in the United States: findings from a supplemental HIV/AIDS surveillance project. *AIDS Education and Prevention, 16*, 440–447.

[34] Yoshioka, M. R., & Schustack, A. (2001). Disclosure of HIV status: Cultural issues of Asian patients. *AIDS Patient Care & STDs, 15*(2), 77–82.

[35] Yoshikawa, H., Wilson, P. A., Hsueh, J., Rosman, E. A., Chin, J., & Kim, J. H. (2003). What front-line CBO staff can tell us about

culturally anchored theories of behavior change in HIV prevention for Asian/Pacific Islanders? *American Journal of Community Psychology, 32*(1-2), 143-58.

[36] Zaidi, I. F., Crepaz, N., Song, R., Wan, C. K., Lin, L. S., Hu, D. J., & Sy, F. S. (2005). Epidemiology of HIV/AIDS among Asians and Pacific Islanders. *AIDS Education and Prevention, 17*, 405–417.

In: Advances in Health and Disease
Editor: Lowell T. Duncan
ISBN: 978-1-53613-020-1
© 2018 Nova Science Publishers, Inc.

Chapter 3

REMOVING HETEROPLASMIC MITOCHONDRIAL DNA MUTATIONS

Juan M. Suárez-Rivero, Marina Villanueva-Paz, Suleva Povea-Cabello, Mario de la Mata, Irene Villalón-García, Mónica Álvarez-Córdoba, David Cotán and José A. Sánchez-Alcázar[1,*]

Centro Andaluz de Biología del Desarrollo (CABD), and Centro de Investigación Biomédica en Red: Enfermedades Raras, Instituto de Salud Carlos III, Universidad Pablo de Olavide-Consejo Superior de Investigaciones Científicas-Junta de Andalucía, Sevilla, Spain

ABSTRACT

Mitochondrial diseases are inborn error disorders caused by total or partial dysfunction of the mitochondrial respiratory chain. These disorders are associated with a wide variety of metabolic and systemic diseases affecting the brain, muscle, heart, retina, optic nerve, liver and endocrine organs. Although many mitochondrial diseases are caused by mutations in the nuclear DNA (nDNA), some of them are due to mutations in the

---

[1*] Corresponding Author E-mail: jasanalc@upo.es.

mitochondrial DNA (mtDNA). As cells contain multiple copies of mtDNA, pathogenic mtDNA mutations frequently coexist with wild-type mtDNA, a phenomenon termed heteroplasmy. Disease phenotypes are only observed once the proportion of wild-type mtDNA drops below a threshold level associated with high accumulations of heteroplasmic mutations. Generally, a critical threshold level above 60-80% of heteroplasmy is required to trigger the oxidative phosphorylation (OXPHOS) defects in specific tissues. Therefore, increasing the proportion of wild-type mtDNA in affected tissues is seen as a viable therapeutic strategy for the treatment of diseases caused by mtDNA mutations.

Nowadays, several heteroplasmy removal/reduction strategies have been proposed (Figure 1). The pharmacologic approach with rapamycin (an autophagy activator) treatment has shown promising results in transmitochondrial cybrid cell lines. Heteroplasmy reduction has been also achieved by the overexpression of mitophagy related proteins such as Parkin. Finally, genome editing via endonucleases, transcription activator-like effector nucleases (TALENs), zinc finger nucleases (ZFNs) and clustered regularly interspaced short palindromic repeats (CRISPR) system represent novel and efficient approaches to treat mitochondrial pathologies in cell models. In this chapter, we will discuss about the advantages and disadvantages of these potential strategies for the treatment of mitochondrial diseases caused by mutant mtDNA.

Keywords: heteroplasmy, mtDNA, treatment, mitochondria

1. INTRODUCTION

Mitochondria are dynamic membranous organelles that have an endosymbiotic origin (Zimorski, Ku, Martin, & Gould, 2014). For this reason, mitochondria still contain their own genetic material (mitochondrial DNA, mtDNA) (R. M. Schwartz & Dayhoff, 1978). Most mitochondrial genes were transferred to the nucleus along evolution, with the exception of 13 protein-coding genes together with two ribosomal RNA and 22 transfer RNA genes (Anderson et al., 1981; Brandvain & Wade, 2009). Mitochondria are involved in several essential cellular processes such as apoptosis (Bhola & Letai, 2016), calcium homeostasis (Finkel et al., 2015) and fatty acid oxidation (Kastaniotis et al., 2017), but their most relevant function is the generation of adenosine triphosphate (ATP) via the oxidative phosphorylation (OXPHOS) system at the inner mitochondrial membrane. The mtDNA-encoded proteins are all subunits of enzyme complexes of the OXPHOS system.

Mutations in mtDNA are relatively rare (1:5000) and are associated with a wide variety of metabolic and systemic diseases affecting the brain, retina, optic nerve, muscle, heart, endocrine organs and liver (Graff, Bui, & Larsson, 2002). Although many mitochondrial diseases are caused by mutations in the nuclear DNA (nDNA), some of them are due to *de novo* or maternally inherited mutations in the mitochondrial genome. As cells contain multiple copies of mtDNA, mutant loci commonly coexist with wild-type ones, a state which is known as heteroplasmy. The opposite term is homoplasmy, meaning that the cells only have one mtDNA haplotype. This determines that mtDNA populations may frequently contain variable proportions of mutant and wild-type mtDNA (Solignac, Monnerot, & Mounolou, 1983). Almost 55% of the reported mtDNA mutations involved in mitochondrial diseases were observed at sites known to be prone to heteroplasmy (Ruiz-Pesini et al., 2007).

Mitochondrial disease phenotypes are only observed once the proportion of wild-type mtDNA drops below a threshold level (Hanna, Nelson, Morgan-Hughes, & Harding, 1995) associated with high accumulations of mtDNA mutations (mitochondrial threshold effect). Generally, heteroplasmy above 60-80% is required to trigger OXPHOS defects in specific tissues (Thorburn & Dahl, 2001). Therefore, increasing the proportion of wild-type mtDNA in affected tissues is seen as a potential therapeutic strategy for the treatment of diseases caused by mtDNA mutations.

Nowadays, several heteroplasmy removal/reduction strategies have been proposed (Figure 1).

The pharmacologic approach with rapamycin (a common anticancer and immunesuppressor compound) treatment has shown promising results in transmitochondrial cybrid cell lines (Dai et al., 2014). Heteroplasmy reduction has also been achieved by overexpression of mitophagy related proteins such as Parkin (Suen, Narendra, Tanaka, Manfredi, & Youle, 2010). Finally, genome editing via endonucleases (Bacman, Williams, Hernandez,

& Moraes, 2007), transcription activator-like effector nucleases (TALENs) (Bacman, Williams, Pinto, Peralta, & Moraes, 2013), zinc finger nucleases (ZFNs) (Gammage, Rorbach, Vincent, Rebar, & Minczuk, 2014) or clustered regularly interspaced short palindromic repeats (CRISPR) system (Jo et al., 2015) represent promising approaches to treat mitochondrial pathologies.

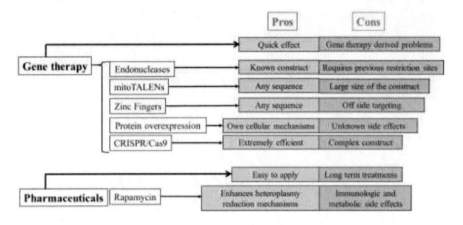

Figure 1. Advantages and disadvantages of heteroplasmy removal/reduction strategies.

2. Heteroplasmy: Mutant *vs* Wild-Type Mitochondrial DNA

The ratio of different types of mtDNAs in a heteroplasmic population may be variable, being usually one mitotype prevalent over the rest of alternative configurations which are present at very low proportions. Generally, the phenotype of the organism is determined by the predominant mtDNA variant (Kmiec, Woloszynska, & Janska, 2006). Furthermore, it has been demonstrated that low levels of heteroplasmy are maternally inherited in humans (Guo et al., 2013).

Heteroplasmy has been related to several disorders such as mitochondrial diseases (Lombes, Aure, Bellanne-Chantelot, Gilleron, & Jardel, 2014), cancer (Qi et al., 2016), diabetes mellitus (Avital et al., 2012) as well as physiological processes such as aging (Sondheimer et al., 2011). Moreover, at least 20% of the population harbors heteroplasmy loads that have been reported to be implicated in several diseases (Ye, Lu, Ma, Keinan, & Gu, 2014). The prevalence of mitochondrial heteroplasmy with high pathogenic potential in healthy individuals, along with the possibility that these mutations may become increasingly frequent within a population of cells across lifespan, emphasizes the importance of managing mitochondrial heteroplasmy to prevent disease progression.

The level of heteroplasmy can vary between cells of the same tissue or organ, from organ to organ within the same person, and between individuals in the same family. Mitochondrial point mutations are usually inherited by the maternal lineage, with multiple individuals in the same family being affected. By contrast, mtDNA deletions are rarely inherited and are never homoplasmic (Chinnery et al., 2004). Homoplasmic mtDNA point mutations usually cause a relatively moderate biochemical defect that typically affects only one organ or tissue (McFarland et al., 2002). On the other hand, heteroplasmic mutations characteristically affect multiple organ systems with high energy requirements such as the nervous system, muscles (including heart) and endocrine organs. The level of heteroplasmy correlates with the extent of organ involvement and therefore with the degree of severity of the clinical phenotype. The biochemical defect is usually severe in affected tissues and requires that mutant mtDNA content exceeds a critical threshold that varies depending on each mutation, tissue, organ and patient. Differences in the levels of heteroplasmy and the precise thresholds are thought to contribute to the characteristic patterns of organ vulnerability observed in different mitochondrial diseases and the clinical heterogeneity observed in patients harboring the same mtDNA mutation.

2.1. Heteroplasmy Origins

The mitochondrial genome has a disproportionately high mutation rate compared to the nuclear genome (Nachman, Brown, Stoneking, & Aquadro, 1996) due to many factors: the lack of a protective chromatin-type packaging of mtDNA, replication errors, insufficient or absent mechanisms of mtDNA repair and high reactive oxygen species (ROS) production in mitochondria. Taken together, all these factors contribute to the continuous creation of new mitotypes.

2.1.1. Spontaneous Mutations in mtDNA

The most commonly believed to be the causes of heteroplasmy are single nucleotide mutations, single base insertions or single base deletions (Stewart & Larsson, 2014). As a result, point mutations, deletions or duplications could be created.

Intracellular ROS are mostly produced in Complex I (CI) and Complex III (CIII) of the mitochondrial respiratory chain (MRC) (Nickel, Kohlhaas, & Maack, 2014). ROS leakage from CIII is thought to have a low impact on mitochondrial matrix components, as it mainly occurs towards the intermembrane space. However, CI is in close proximity or even in contact with the mtDNA due to its localization on the internal surface of the inner membrane. Therefore Complex I-derived ROS are thought to have the highest impact on oxidative damage to DNA. As a consequence, 8-oxo-7, 8-dihydro-2′deoxyguanosine (8-oxodG) is one of the most abundant mutations caused by the oxidative conversion of guanosine. In agreement with this hypothesis, guanosine oxidative damage accumulation rate in mtDNA is higher than in nDNA, suggesting that mitochondrial genome is more affected by ROS than nuclear genome (Lauri, Pompilio, & Capogrossi, 2014). The ROS-induced mt-DNA mutations, if not quickly repaired, are propagated and fixed at each mtDNA replication cycle. In fact, during replication, 8-oxodG is paired with an adenine instead of cytosine, which results in a G→T point mutation. Furthermore, oxidized cytosine, another ROS-induced mutation, is mispaired with adenine, resulting in C→A mutations (Wang, Kreutzer, & Essigmann, 1998).

The frequency of somatic mtDNA mutations can exceed the mutation frequency of the nuclear genome by several orders of magnitude (Brown, George, & Wilson, 1979). Although this difference could be explained by mtDNA damage due to elevated concentrations of ROS, recent studies argue against any significant contribution of oxidative damage in mtDNA mutation appearance (Itsara et al., 2014). Most of the mutations detected are transition mutations and not the G→T transversion usually related to ROS damage. In fact, current whole genome analysis by next-generation sequencing techniques shows misincorporations by the mitochondrial DNA polymerase γ or deamination of cytidine and adenosine as the primary mutagenic events in mtDNA (Kennedy, Salk, Schmitt, & Loeb, 2013). These mutation patterns indicate that replication errors by mitochondrial DNA polymerase γ and/or spontaneous base hydrolysis are responsible for the bulk of accumulated point mutations in mtDNA.

2.1.2. Paternal mtDNA Leakage

In animals, mitochondrial genomes are mostly maternally inherited, with only a few exceptions showing paternal transmission or biparental inheritance (Ladoukakis & Zouros, 2001). However, it has been proven that heteroplasmy can be produced by occasional paternal mtDNA leakage (paternal mtDNA contribution to progeny) (Aksyonova et al., 2005; Morgan et al., 2013). Paternal leakage of mtDNA is highly penalized because it may lead to further rearrangements, since the mtDNAs passed down from males and females could recombine promoting the appearance of new mutations (Ladoukakis & Zouros, 2001). Nowadays, only a few cases of paternal mtDNA transmission are reported in humans (M. Schwartz & Vissing, 2002).

Paternal leakage may result from a failure in mitonuclear mechanisms that normally maintain maternal mtDNA inheritance. In these cases the paternally derived mtDNA is assumed to be extremely diluted in comparison with the maternal mtDNA. Several studies suggest that paternal leakage is more common than it is believed, although it is barely detectable (Wolff & Gemmell, 2008). This biparental inherence of mtDNA could have almost no effect due to the mtDNA bottleneck transmission during embryogenesis. This bottleneck phenomenon is caused by the fact that only a subset of all embryo cells and consequently mtDNAs present in the zygote will ultimately contribute properly to the embryo itself (Fleming, Javed, & Hay, 1992). As the number of mitochondria in these embryonic cells is low, rare mtDNA haplotypes such as the paternally transmitted mtDNA are likely to be lost if present at low frequencies in the zygote.

2.1.3. mtDNA Recombination

Enzymes involved in homologous recombination have been identified in mammalian mitochondria (Thyagarajan, Padua, & Campbell, 1996), however heteroplasmy of animal mtDNA driven by recombination has been only rarely described (Piganeau, Gardner, & Eyre-Walker, 2004). In humans, the most direct evidence came from a patient who suffered a mitochondrial myopathy with a 10:1 ratio of paternal to maternal mtDNA in his skeletal muscle. A deletion in his paternally inherited mtDNA gave rise to the disorder. It was found that 0.7% of mtDNA molecules were recombinant (Kraytsberg et al., 2004).

Recombination can occur between heterologous mitochondrial molecules harboring pathogenic mutations (D'Aurelio et al., 2004). In addition, studies on the patterns of tetraplasmy in doubly heteroplasmic individuals not only suggest that mitochondrial recombination is relatively common in human skeletal muscle tissue but also demonstrate the inheritability of recombinant mtDNA molecules (Zsurka et al., 2005). In order to have a real repercussion on the cell, recombination must occur between two different mitotypes; therefore, a previous state of mitochondrial heteroplasmy is required. In fact, some mitochondrial rearrangements could be found at a very low level in healthy human tissues as a result of recombination but with no pathological consequences (Kajander et al., 2000). These alterations in the mtDNA genome are called sublimons, and they refer to low-abundance, rearranged mtDNAs, that are structurally similar to the multiple rearranged mtDNAs found in patients with mitochondrial disorders. Sublimons were found to be scattered around the mitochondrial genome, but several hotspot regions were detected (Kajander, Karhunen, & Jacobs, 2002). It has been hypothesized that these rearrangements may facilitate the rate of recombination and give rise to new mitotypes.

2.2. Heteroplasmy Expansion

All mtDNA mutations are originated within a single organelle, inside a single cell. Keeping in mind that each cell contains hundreds to thousands mtDNA molecules, a single molecule containing a mutation lies well below the mutation-detection threshold for most current technologies. There are some hypotheses which claim that a mutation affecting one molecule can eventually reach a high frequency within a population of cells and thereby be detected. In this chapter, we will focus on mitochondrial related mechanisms of heteroplasmy expansion, bearing in mind that there are nuclear factors behind this phenomenon that can generate a higher level of complexity.

2.2.1. Vegetative Segregation of mtDNA

When a cell divides, the mtDNA molecules pass randomly to the daughter cells. If there is a heteroplasmic variant present then, by chance, each daughter cell can receive a different proportion of mutant mtDNA. This process is called vegetative segregation and provides an explanation to the observed changes in the level of heteroplasmy of dividing cells. Statistically, for neutral genetic variants, the overall mutation level will remain constant in an infinite population; but, in a finite pool of dividing cells, the mutation level can drift up or down through random genetic drift. However, if a mutation has a severe effect on cell function and/or prevents the replication of the cell, then selection against the mutation will occur at the cellular level. This negative selection is thought to be the reason why levels of some pathogenic mitochondrial mutations decrease during life (Rajasimha, Chinnery, & Samuels, 2008). In cell culture studies, different mtDNA mutations can drift in either direction or the overall heteroplasmy level can remain stable (Lehtinen et al., 2000). The reason why a mutation can drift up, down or remain stable in different cell lines is yet unknown but is thought that nuclear genes may influence the segregation pattern (Raap et al., 2012).

In some specific cases, antiretroviral drugs may interfere with the mitochondrial DNA polymerase γ activity, reducing temporally the mtDNA content which could create a genetic bottleneck with the mutant mtDNA, leading to a clonal expansion of the mutation (Payne et al., 2011). Finally, it is believed that shorter mitochondrial genomes (with large deletions) could have a replicative advantage versus wild-type mtDNA due to a reduced replication time, however, *in silico* models have concluded that this process would almost need a century to surpass the wild-type mtDNA and reach the critical heteroplasmy threshold (Kowald, Dawson, & Kirkwood, 2014).

2.2.2. Impairment of Mitochondrial Dynamics

Mitochondria are very versatile organelles which carry out continuous fusion and fission processes in response to various cellular signals. Mitochondrial dynamics, including mitochondrial fission/fusion, movements and turnover, are essential for the mitochondrial network quality control. Mitophagy is the process by which dysfunctional or damaged mitochondria are selectively targeted by autophagosomes and delivered to lysosomes in order to be recycled by the cell. Mitochondrial homeostasis requires a perfect equilibrium between mitophagy and mitochondrial biogenesis. Mitophagy also requires the defective mitochondria to be isolated from the mitochondrial network through mitochondrial fission. Thus, balancing fission and fusion is crucial for both, mixing mtDNA genomes which allows functional complementation and for promoting the mitophagic elimination of mitochondria with excessive mutant mtDNA, and therefore modulating its possible clonal expansion (Carelli et al., 2015).

Alterations in mitochondrial dynamics could lead to a loss of homeostasis in the mitochondrial network impairing the selection against mutant mtDNA. Several studies have shown that alterations in the mitochondrial fusion proteins like mitofusins (MFN1 and MFN2) (Chen et al., 2010; Rouzier et al., 2012) or mitophagy proteins (Villanueva Paz et al., 2016) can modify the heteroplasmy load through time. Furthermore, in *Caenorhabditis elegans*, mitochondrial unfolded protein response (UPR^{mt}) allows the mutant mtDNA molecules to accumulate by reducing mitophagy (Gitschlag et al., 2016).

Autophagy processes, including mitophagy, are compromised during aging and therefore, they may contribute to age-associated pathologies including neurodegeneration and the appearance of mitochondrial diseases (Martinez-Lopez, Athonvarangkul, & Singh, 2015).

2.2.3. Randomness in Mitochondrial Segregation

MtDNA is being continuously destroyed and replicated, even in non-dividing cells, by a process termed relaxed replication. In a heteroplasmic cell, it is possible that, by chance, a variant molecule might be replicated more frequently than the wild-type molecule, leading to a change in the overall heteroplasmy level within the cell. Bioinformatics models have shown that, in a fixed population of cells, this random process can lead to significant changes in heteroplasmy levels which progressively increase with the cell life span. These results provide one explanation for the apparent clonal expansion of specific mtDNA molecules during human life (Chinnery & Samuels, 1999) and could explain why a huge percentage of mitochondrial patients are diagnosed among elderly people (Elson, Samuels, Turnbull, & Chinnery, 2001).

Even though it seems to work *in silico* models, the heteroplasmy expansion hypothesis goes against the cellular mechanisms to maintain a healthy mitochondrial network such as mitophagy. Generally, defective mitochondria tend to lose their membrane potential allowing Parkin and the rest of mitophagy-involved proteins to be recruited (Ding & Yin, 2012), hence reducing the adverse effects of relaxed replication. On the other hand, it is known that mitophagy declines during aging, triggering a loss of homeostasis that would enable mitochondrial mutations to rise over their basal levels (Lipinski et al., 2010).

3. MITOCHONDRIAL GENE THERAPY

One interesting fact about heteroplasmy and its threshold effects is that a reduction in the pathological phenotype can be achieved without completely removing mutant alleles. Thanks to the wild-type mtDNA compensating effect, we could treat the pathology by simply reducing the levels of the mutant allele below threshold levels (Bacman et al., 2013).

Therefore, heteroplasmy shift is an attractive strategy for the genetic therapy of mtDNA disorders. Thus, all of the genetic approaches are based on the elimination of the mutant mtDNA. Once the mutant mtDNA is degraded, its copy number control ensures that the residual (wild-type) intact mitochondrial genomes repopulate the cell (Diaz et al., 2002).

3.1. Nucleases

In cases at which the mitochondrial mutation corresponds to a recognition site of a restriction enzyme (RE) it could be possible to develop a mitochondria-targeted enzyme. Due to the bacterial origin of restriction enzymes, a specific construct is needed. To design a mitochondrial-targeted endonuclease, the coding gene is "mammalianized" with the addition of a human COX8A N-terminal mitochondrial localization signal to direct the enzyme to mitochondria. Recognition and cleavage by the enzyme lead to a reduction in the relative level of the target allele, a mutant mtDNA in our case, through cleavage-stimulated mtDNA degradation. Thus, only the uncleaved mtDNA or wild-type mtDNA can replicate and restore normal mtDNA levels as well as optimize the OXPHOS function (Bayona-Bafaluy, Blits, Battersby, Shoubridge, & Moraes, 2005).

A rodent mouse–rat cybrid cell line containing both mouse and rat mtDNA was the first cell line used to demonstrate the efficacy of the REs (Srivastava & Moraes, 2001). Mouse mtDNA contained two *Pst*I sites while rat mtDNA contained none. After the expression of variant *Pst*I targeted to mitochondria (mito-*Pst*I) a significant shift in the relative abundance of rat versus mouse mtDNA was achieved, proving the efficacy of mitochondria-targeted endonucleases for mtDNA heteroplasmy shift. In human cells, this technique was used in a cybrid cell line carrying the heteroplasmic mutation m.8993T>C, related to Leigh and NARP (neuropathy, ataxia, and retinitis pigmentosa) syndromes, which creates a *Sma*I restriction site (Tanaka et al., 2002). Complete elimination of m.8993T>C and restoration of ATP levels were achieved after five cycles of transfection and selection of cybrids with an initial mutation load of 98% after using a *Sma*I mitochondria targeted variant.

REs have also been tested in mouse oocytes and one-cell embryos. The model was a heteroplasmic BALB/NZB mouse germline that carries both the BALB and NZB wild-type mtDNA haplotypes. The BALB haplotype contains an *Apa*LI restriction site that is missing in the NZB haplotype. A mitochondria-targeted form of the enzyme was created (mito- *Apa*LI) and by its expression, cells derived from these mice enabled examination of the transient depletion and kinetics of heteroplasmy shift. The mtDNA depletion was found to correlate with certain initial levels of the target BALB mtDNA and repletion was complete in one cell cycle (Reddy et al., 2015). This approach was used in mouse tissues via injection of the construct in brain and muscle cells using adenovirus type 5 vector and it was proved to be translatable to animal models (Bayona-Bafaluy et al., 2005). The ability to induce heteroplasmy shift in specific tissues has also been demonstrated using cardiotropic adeno-associated virus type 6 (AAV6) and hepatotropic Ad5 to deliver mito-*Apa*LI (Bacman et al., 2007).

Although REs-targeted mitochondria have been reported to change mtDNA heteroplasmy, their clinical application is limited due to the fact that only a few mtDNA mutations create restriction sites. To solve this limitation, there are endonucleases with modular DNA recognition domains, which can be designed to target almost any sequence. Nowadays the most promising systems available with these characteristics are TALENs and ZFNs.

3.2. TALENs

TALENs are made of DNA-binding modules fused to a nuclease domain from a *Fok*I restriction enzyme. The DNA-binding specificity of TALEN domains is given by tandem copies of 34 amino acid repeats that bind preferentially to one of the four DNA bases depending on the aminoacid which is placed at the 12th or 13th position of each of the repeats. The nucleotide affinity of these repeat variable di-residues is well understood, providing the basis to engineering novel specificities (Moscou &

Bogdanove, 2009). A particular feature of the system is that TALENs work as heterodimers, requiring two TALEN monomers to bind closely spaced DNA sequences, allowing their *Fok*I nuclease domains to dimerize and cleave DNA (Cermak et al., 2011). Despite TALEN can be very specific, this specificity is not perfect and off-site cleavages, in large and complex genomes, can be an issue (Watanabe et al., 2012). The high specificity of TALENs is due to its molecular activity via the combination of both, sequence specificity of TALEN binding and the positional requirements of *Fok*I cleavage. Those TALENs designed exclusively to target the mitochondria are called "mitoTALENs" and include a mitochondrial localization signal (for instance, *SOD2* or *COX8A/Su9*). MitoTALENs work as endonucleases producing a double-strand break point in the sequence followed by a quick degradation.

MitoTALENs have been used to induce heteroplasmy shift in several cell models of mitochondrial diseases. Patient-derived cybrids are the most popular cell model to test this kind of technique due to their advantages in mitochondrial diseases research (Dunn, Cannon, Irwin, & Pinkert, 2012). MERRF (myoclonic epilepsy with ragged red fibers, mt.8344A>G) and Leigh syndrome (mt.13513G>A) cybrids, harboring about 80% of mutant mtDNA, which were transfected with its respective mitoTALENs showed a robust change in heteroplasmy up to 80% of wild-type mtDNA. This variation not only affects mtDNA content but the general OXPHOS function (Hashimoto et al., 2015). In another study using cybrids with the Leber's hereditary optic neuropathy with dystonia (LHON, mt.14459G>A) point mutation, mitoTALENs were able to induce a shift of wild-type mtDNA content from 10% to 90% (Bacman et al., 2013). However, mitoTALENs are not only restricted to point mutations; they have been also used to treat mitochondrial deletions. The mtDNA deletion m.8483_13459del4977 is the most common deletion being present in approximately 30% of all patients with mtDNA deletions as well as during aging (Corral-Debrinski et al., 1992; Schon et al., 1989). Δ5–mitoTALEN is a variant construct which can degrade DNA sequences suffering deletions instead of mutations. As well as any other TALEN, it is composed by two monomers that bind specifically to target sequences, but only in the deletion mutant mtDNA the monomers are close enough to promote FokI dimerization and cleavage. This TALEN assay showed that the Δ5–mitoTALEN was effective in reducing the mtDNA deletion load and changing mtDNA heteroplasmy towards a predominance of wild–type mtDNA (Bacman et al., 2013). Surprisingly, mitoTALENs only take about 2 to 3 days to switch the heteroplasmy ratios in most cases.

MitoTALENs have also been used in mouse NZB/BALB oocytes for the specific elimination of NZB mtDNA. The same methods to those explained in the previous endonucleases section were used for such purpose. MtDNA content analysis 48 h after NZB mito-TALEN mRNA injection demonstrated the specific decrease of NZB mtDNA and a consequential increase of the relative BALB mtDNA levels (Reddy et al., 2015). These results prove the potential of designed mito-TALENs for the specific elimination of mutant mtDNA in the germline to prevent the transmission of mitochondrial diseases.

Although mitoTALENs are promising tools for gene therapy, they show a technical problem related to the large size of the construct (requires two monomers) that makes difficult their packaging in current vector systems However, this would not be an obstacle in certain mitoTALENs since the complexity of mt-DNA is much lower than that of the nuclear genome.Thus, smaller TALEN DNA-binding domains would still be effective in shifting heteroplasmy without increasing off-site cleavage (Hashimoto et al., 2015). Eventually, some vectors could cause non desirable side effects, as observed in gene therapy procedures.

3.3. ZFNs

The Cys_2His_2 class of ZFNs has been proven to be particularly effective for engineering customized DNA binding proteins with high specificity and affinity for a given DNA sequence. They have been previously used to alter nuclear gene expression by modifying DNA in a sequence-specific manner (Cohn et al., 2007; Falke & Juliano, 2003). Cys_2–His_2 zinc-finger domains as used in ZFNs are small 34-amino acid protein motifs containing an antiparallel β-sheet and an α-helix stabilized by a zinc ion. Each domain binds a triplet DNA sequence and combinations of zinc-finger domains can be designed to bind many specific sequences. The addition of C-terminal *Fok*I nuclease domain and the design of pairs of proteins that bind DNA in close tail-tail proximity enable the cleavage of DNA at specific sequences. ZFNs are predominantly DNA binding proteins adapted to operate in the nucleus. Even in the absence of nuclear localization signals they are often located in the nucleus (Papworth, Kolasinska, & Minczuk, 2006). In order to use designed ZFNs to manipulate mtDNA, they have to be both, effectively targeted to mitochondria and, at the same time, excluded from the nucleus to prevent their undesired binding to nuclear DNA, which could be harmful (Papworth et al., 2003). To overcome this and at the same time enable efficient trafficking to mitochondria, it is necessary to incorporate nuclear export sequences into ZFN monomers (Minczuk, Papworth, Kolasinska, Murphy, & Klug, 2006).

ZFNs technology has been used to target pathogenic mitochondrial genomes in cybrid cells, such as those harboring the mutation mt.8993T>G (Leigh's syndrome) (Gammage et al., 2014) or the deletion m.8483_13459del4977 (Minczuk et al., 2006). Aiming to reduce off-site cleavage, almost all recombinant nucleases utilize the hetero-dimeric *Fok*I domains (Doyon et al., 2011). These domains have modified protein sequences that create a different dimerization face on each monomer and prevent dimerization of identical monomers. This modification has been found to carry out a 100-fold reduction of self-self dimerization.

The current standard modality of ZFN therapy delivery is through recombinant adeno-associated virus (AAV), and tissue-specific serotypes thereof. Although the AAV is generally considered to be a transient, non-integrating genetic vector, it has been shown in animal models that viral genomes persist, in an episomal state, for essentially the entire life-span of the lab animal, most reliably in post-mitotic or slowly-dividing tissues (Mingozzi & High, 2011). In conclusion, a fine level of control over these designed enzymes will be essential for achieving any successful therapeutic outcome.

3.4. CRISPR/Cas9

Despite the huge potential of mitoTALEN and ZFNs-mediated mtDNA editing, more user-friendly and efficient alternative methods are necessary to overcome difficulties in mtDNA modification either for correction of dysfunctional mtDNA or for producing dysfunctional mtDNA in order to create mitochondria-associated disease models. The CRISPR/Cas9 system has been widely used for nuclear DNA editing to generate mutations or correct specific disease alleles. The mitochondrial targeting sequence of subunit VIII of human cytochrome c oxidase has been attached to mitoCas9 construct for mitochondrial delivery. MitoCas9 robustly localize at mitochondria together with the single guide RNA (sgRNA) targeting the COX3 mitochondrial gene and it is able to cleavage 80% of total mtDNA, which demonstrates its functional application for mtDNA editing (Jo et al., 2015). These results prove the successful application of CRISPR/Cas9 in mitochondrial genome editing and suggest the possibility for *in vitro* and *in vivo* manipulation of mtDNA in a site-specific manner.

Although CRISPR/Cas9 is a relatively recent technique, mitochondria-targeting Cas9 combined with mtDNA-specific sgRNA provides an opportunity to generate homoplasmic or heteroplasmic mutant mtDNA strains, repairing mutant models and therefore, being an extremely specific therapeutic approach.

3.5. Protein Overexpression

Mitophagy is the process by which dysfunctional or damaged mitochondria are selectively targeted by autophagosomes and delivered to lysosomes to be recycled by the cell. The most characterized mechanism regulating the recruitment of autophagosomes towards mitochondria is that driven by phosphatase and tensin homolog (PTEN)-induced putative kinase 1 (PINK1) and Parkin (Youle & Narendra, 2011). Mutations in the PINK1 and Parkin genes are well known causes of autosomal recessive forms of Parkinson's disease, and numerous studies associate this to the role of these proteins in mitochondrial quality control (Pickrell & Youle, 2015). Parkin can translocate to depolarized mitochondria and activate their elimination by autophagy suggesting that it may function in the mitochondrial quality control (Narendra, Tanaka, Suen, & Youle, 2008).

Recent studies have shown that Parkin overexpression has the capacity to selectively eliminate mitochondria containing high levels of COXI mutant mtDNA (Suen et al., 2010). Heteroplasmic cybrids shifted its wild-type mtDNA from 20% to 90% in a period of 200 days and restored most of the mitochondrial function. These results support the hypothesis that Parkin may normally select wild-type mtDNA by mediating the elimination of dysfunctional mitochondria containing mutant mtDNA. Loss or impaired Parkin function may cause excessive accumulation of deleterious mutant mtDNA. In addition, it could indicate that endogenous Parkin levels may be limiting for the negative selection of dysfunctional mitochondria in at least some cell types, and that up-regulation of Parkin expression may be therapeutically beneficial for hereditary and somatically acquired mitochondrial diseases.

From the point of view of mitochondrial recombination, many mutations in mtDNA take the form of large-scale rearrangements, either partial deletions or tandem duplications (Holt et al., 1989). Duplications can co-exist with deletions (Poulton et al., 1993), and intramolecular homologous recombination of partially duplicated mtDNA could produce a wild-type monomer and a partially deleted mtDNA molecule (Dunbar et al., 1993). The Holliday junction resolvase or cruciform cutting endonuclease (CCE1) has a crucial function for mtDNA stability in yeasts (Kleff, Kemper, & Sternglanz, 1992). Despite there is no known homologue of CCE1 in the human genome, its expression in human cybrids carrying partial duplications shifted the wild-type mtDNA content from ~15% to ~75% (Sembongi, Di Re, Bokori-Brown, & Holt, 2007). This procedure led to the selection of lower order rearrangements and wild-type mtDNA, suggesting that the yeast enzyme is capable of mediating homologue recombination in human mitochondria. This approach was conceived as a potential therapeutic strategy. However sustained expression of high levels of CCE1 provokes mtDNA depletion, and therefore it is necessary to strictly control this gene's expression to select and maintain wild-type mtDNA.

4. TARGETING HETEROPLASMY WITH PHARMACOLOGICAL TREATMENTS

As mentioned before, mitophagy has a preferential degradation activity for dysfunctional mitochondria. In cells with a heteroplasmic pathogenic mtDNA mutation, after mitochondrial fission, a separated mitochondrion with high mutant mtDNA content will be less likely to maintain its membrane potential and more likely to produce elevated ROS, increasing the probability of being targeted by mitophagy (Wei, Liu, & Chen, 2015). Therefore, enhancing the mitophagy or fission pathways could promote the elimination of defective mitochondria.

This strategy has been examined by using rapamycin, an autophagy activator, in cybrids harboring the LHON mutation mt.11778G>A (Dai et al., 2014). Rapamycin treatment for 20 weeks reduced the mutational load up to 95%. To assess whether mtDNA mutation levels would increase again in the absence of rapamycin, cells were incubated for 4 additional weeks without the treatment. The withdrawal of rapamycin resulted in a return of the 12% to the 29% of mtDNA mutation levels.

The rapamycin-sensitive mTORC1 (mammalian target of rapamycin complex 1) has proved to be essential for the regulation of protein translation and autophagy (Kim & Guan, 2015). Treatment with rapamycin inhibits mTORC1 and promotes autophagy, even in the presence of nutrients. However, it has potentially serious side effects in humans, including glucose intolerance and immunosuppression which may preclude the long-term use of rapamycin as a therapy for mitochondrial diseases. However, a recent study has evidenced that an intermittent dosing schedule compared to daily treatment reduces the effects of rapamycin on glucose tolerance and immune system (Arriola Apelo et al., 2016). Furthermore, FDA-approved rapamycin analogs (everolimus and temsirolimus) have been proven to efficiently inhibit mTORC1 without unwanted side effects. These results suggest that adverse side effects of rapamycin treatment can be mitigated through intermittent dosing or the use of rapamycin analogs (Arriola Apelo et al., 2016).

CONCLUSION

Heteroplasmic mtDNA mutations cause a group of disorders with a great variety of symptoms which depends, among others, on the nuclear background, type of mutation, mutant mtDNA levels, affected tissue and age. This makes it extremely difficult to develop a universal treatment for these disorders. However, most therapeutic options share the common strategy of targeting the subpopulation of defective mitochondria. Currently, gene therapy has mainly been applied to cellular models of mitochondrial diseases. However, it is difficult to directly compare the efficacy of these methods due to the heterogeneity of cell lines and functional outcome assays used in these studies. In addition, the main challenges for its acceptability are the unpredictable toxic effects caused by the immunogenicity of delivery vectors and their uncontrollable integration at inappropriate sites that may lead to the oncogenic transformation of the host cells.

Pharmacological treatment could be another promising strategy. However, few studies examining the effect of drugs on heteroplasmy levels in cellular models haven been undertaken.

In this review, we have discussed the efficacy of several approaches, but it is necessary to establish common criteria for their evaluation such as cellular models, metabolic or functional outcome parameters as well as to assess the adverse secondary effects. Finally, the next step would be to test potential treatments in animal models. In fact, one of the most challenging problems of the current mitochondrial therapy research is the lack of such genetic models for mtDNA-related disorders.

REFERENCES

Aksyonova, E., Sinyavskaya, M., Danilenko, N., Pershina, L., Nakamura, C., & Davydenko, O. (2005). Heteroplasmy and paternally oriented shift of the organellar DNA composition in barley-wheat hybrids during backcrosses with wheat parents. *Genome, 48*, 761-769.

Anderson, S., Bankier, A. T., Barrell, B. G., de Bruijn, M. H., Coulson, A. R., Drouin, J., ... Young, I. G. (1981). Sequence and organization of the human mitochondrial genome. *Nature, 290*(5806), 457-465.

Arriola Apelo, S. I., Neuman, J. C., Baar, E. L., Syed, F. A., Cummings, N. E., Brar, H. K., ... Lamming, D. W. (2016). Alternative rapamycin treatment regimens mitigate the impact of rapamycin on glucose homeostasis and the immune system. *Aging cell, 15*, 28-38.

Avital, G., Buchshtav, M., Zhidkov, I., Tuval Feder, J., Dadon, S., Rubin, E., ... Mishmar, D. (2012). Mitochondrial DNA heteroplasmy in diabetes and normal adults: role of acquired and inherited mutational patterns in twins. *Hum Mol Genet, 21*(19), 4214-4224. doi: 10.1093/hmg/dds245.

Bacman, S. R., Williams, S. L., Hernandez, D., & Moraes, C. T. (2007). Modulating mtDNA heteroplasmy by mitochondria-targeted restriction endonucleases in a 'differential multiple cleavage-site' model. [Research Support, N.I.H., Extramural]. *Gene Ther, 14*(18), 1309-1318.

Bacman, S. R., Williams, S. L., Pinto, M., Peralta, S., & Moraes, C. T. (2013). Specific elimination of mutant mitochondrial genomes in patient-derived cells by mitoTALENs. *Nat Med, 19*(9), 1111-1113. doi: 10.1038/nm.3261.

Bayona-Bafaluy, M. P., Blits, B., Battersby, B. J., Shoubridge, E. A., & Moraes, C. T. (2005). Rapid directional shift of mitochondrial DNA heteroplasmy in animal tissues by a mitochondrially targeted restriction endonuclease. *Proc Natl Acad Sci U S A, 102*(40), 14392-14397.

Bhola, P. D., & Letai, A. (2016). Mitochondria-Judges and Executioners of Cell Death Sentences. *Molecular cell, 61*, 695-704.

Brandvain, Y., & Wade, M. J. (2009). The functional transfer of genes from the mitochondria to the nucleus: the effects of selection, mutation, population size and rate of self-fertilization. *Genetics, 182*(4), 1129-1139.

Brown, W. M., George, M., Jr., & Wilson, A. C. (1979). Rapid evolution of animal mitochondrial DNA. *Proc Natl Acad Sci U S A, 76*(4), 1967-1971.

Carelli, V., Maresca, A., Caporali, L., Trifunov, S., Zanna, C., & Rugolo, M. (2015). Mitochondria: Biogenesis and mitophagy balance in segregation and clonal expansion of mitochondrial DNA mutations. *The international journal of biochemistry & cell biology, 63*, 21-24.

Cermak, T., Doyle, E. L., Christian, M., Wang, L., Zhang, Y., Schmidt, C., ... Voytas, D. F. (2011). Efficient design and assembly of custom TALEN and other TAL effector-based constructs for DNA targeting. *Nucleic Acids Res, 39*(12), e82.

Cohn, A. C., Toomes, C., Potter, C., Towns, K. V., Hewitt, A. W., Inglehearn, C. F., ... Mackey, D. A. (2007). Autosomal dominant optic atrophy: penetrance and expressivity in patients with OPA1 mutations. *Am J Ophthalmol, 143*(4), 656-662.

Corral-Debrinski, M., Horton, T., Lott, M. T., Shoffner, J. M., Beal, M. F., & Wallace, D. C. (1992). Mitochondrial DNA deletions in human brain: regional variability and increase with advanced age.. *Nat Genet, 2*(4), 324-329.

Chen, H., Vermulst, M., Wang, Y. E., Chomyn, A., Prolla, T. A., McCaffery, J. M., & Chan, D. C. (2010). Mitochondrial fusion is required for mtDNA stability in skeletal muscle and tolerance of mtDNA mutations. *Cell, 141*(2), 280-289.

Chinnery, P. F., DiMauro, S., Shanske, S., Schon, E. A., Zeviani, M., Mariotti, C., ... Turnbull, D. M. (2004). Risk of developing a mitochondrial DNA deletion disorder. *Lancet, 364*(9434), 592-596.

Chinnery, P. F., & Samuels, D. C. (1999). Relaxed replication of mtDNA: A model with implications for the expression of disease. *Am J Hum Genet, 64*(4), 1158-1165.

D'Aurelio, M., Gajewski, C. D., Lin, M. T., Mauck, W. M., Shao, L. Z., Lenaz, G., ... Manfredi, G. (2004). Heterologous mitochondrial DNA recombination in human cells. *Hum Mol Genet, 13*(24), 3171-3179.

Dai, Y., Zheng, K., Clark, J., Swerdlow, R. H., Pulst, S. M., Sutton, J. P., ... Simon, D. K. (2014). Rapamycin drives selection against a pathogenic heteroplasmic mitochondrial DNA mutation. *Hum Mol Genet, 23*(3), 637-647.

Diaz, F., Bayona-Bafaluy, M. P., Rana, M., Mora, M., Hao, H., & Moraes, C. T. (2002). Human mitochondrial DNA with large deletions repopulates organelles faster than full-length genomes under relaxed copy number control. *Nucleic Acids Res, 30*(21), 4626-4633.

Ding, W. X., & Yin, X. M. (2012). Mitophagy: mechanisms, pathophysiological roles, and analysis. *Biol Chem, 393*(7), 547-564.

Doyon, Y., Vo, T. D., Mendel, M. C., Greenberg, S. G., Wang, J., Xia, D. F., ... Holmes, M. C. (2011). Enhancing zinc-finger-nuclease activity with improved obligate heterodimeric architectures. *Nat Methods, 8*(1), 74-79.

Dunbar, D. R., Moonie, P. A., Swingler, R. J., Davidson, D., Roberts, R., & Holt, I. J. (1993). Maternally transmitted partial direct tandem duplication of mitochondrial DNA associated with diabetes mellitus. *Hum Mol Genet, 2*(10), 1619-1624.

Dunn, D. A., Cannon, M. V., Irwin, M. H., & Pinkert, C. A. (2012). Animal models of human mitochondrial DNA mutations. [Review]. *Biochim Biophys Acta, 1820*(5), 601-607.

Elson, J. L., Samuels, D. C., Turnbull, D. M., & Chinnery, P. F. (2001). Random intracellular drift explains the clonal expansion of mitochondrial DNA mutations with age. *Am J Hum Genet, 68*(3), 802-806.

Falke, D., & Juliano, R. L. (2003). Selective gene regulation with designed transcription factors: implications for therapy. *Curr Opin Mol Ther, 5*(2), 161-166.

Finkel, T., Menazza, S., Holmstrom, K. M., Parks, R. J., Liu, J., Sun, J., ... Murphy, E. (2015). The ins and outs of mitochondrial calcium. *Circ Res, 116*(11), 1810-1819.

Fleming, T. P., Javed, Q., & Hay, M. (1992). Epithelial differentiation and intercellular junction formation in the mouse early embryo. *Dev Suppl*, 105-112.

Gammage, P. A., Rorbach, J., Vincent, A. I., Rebar, E. J., & Minczuk, M. (2014). Mitochondrially targeted ZFNs for selective degradation of pathogenic mitochondrial genomes bearing large-scale deletions or point mutations. *EMBO Mol Med, 6*(4), 458-466.

Gitschlag, B. L., Kirby, C. S., Samuels, D. C., Gangula, R. D., Mallal, S. A., & Patel, M. R. (2016). Homeostatic Responses Regulate Selfish Mitochondrial Genome Dynamics in C. elegans. *Cell Metab, 24*(1), 91-103.

Graff, C., Bui, T. H., & Larsson, N. G. (2002). Mitochondrial diseases. [Review]. *Best Pract Res Clin Obstet Gynaecol, 16*(5), 715-728.

Guo, Y., Li, C. I., Sheng, Q., Winther, J. F., Cai, Q., Boice, J. D., & Shyr, Y. (2013). Very low-level heteroplasmy mtDNA variations are inherited in humans. *J Genet Genomics, 40*(12), 607-615.

Hanna, M. G., Nelson, I. P., Morgan-Hughes, J. A., & Harding, A. E. (1995). Impaired mitochondrial translation in human myoblasts harbouring the mitochondrial DNA tRNA lysine 8344 A-->G (MERRF) mutation: relationship to proportion of mutant mitochondrial DNA. *J Neurol Sci, 130*(2), 154-160.

Hashimoto, M., Bacman, S. R., Peralta, S., Falk, M. J., Chomyn, A., Chan, D. C., ... Moraes, C. T. (2015). MitoTALEN: A General Approach to Reduce Mutant mtDNA Loads and Restore Oxidative Phosphorylation Function in Mitochondrial Diseases. *Mol Ther, 23*(10), 1592-1599.

Holt, I. J., Harding, A. E., Cooper, J. M., Schapira, A. H., Toscano, A., Clark, J. B., & Morgan-Hughes, J. A. (1989). Mitochondrial myopathies: clinical and biochemical features of 30 patients with major deletions of muscle mitochondrial DNA. *Ann Neurol, 26*(6), 699-708.

Itsara, L. S., Kennedy, S. R., Fox, E. J., Yu, S., Hewitt, J. J., Sanchez-Contreras, M., ... Pallanck, L. J. (2014). Oxidative stress is not a major contributor to somatic mitochondrial DNA mutations. *PLoS Genet, 10*(2), e1003974.

Jo, A., Ham, S., Lee, G. H., Lee, Y. I., Kim, S., Lee, Y. S., ... Lee, Y. (2015). Efficient Mitochondrial Genome Editing by CRISPR/Cas9. [Research Support, Non-U.S. Gov't]. *Biomed Res Int, 2015*, 305716.

Kajander, O. A., Karhunen, P. J., & Jacobs, H. T. (2002). The relationship between somatic mtDNA rearrangements, human heart disease and aging. *Hum Mol Genet, 11*(3), 317-324.

Kajander, O. A., Rovio, A. T., Majamaa, K., Poulton, J., Spelbrink, J. N., Holt, I. J., ... Jacobs, H. T. (2000). Human mtDNA sublimons resemble rearranged mitochondrial genoms found in pathological states. *Hum Mol Genet, 9*(19), 2821-2835.

Kastaniotis, A. J., Autio, K. J., Keratar, J. M., Monteuuis, G., Makela, A. M., Nair, R. R., ... Hiltunen, J. K. (2017). Mitochondrial fatty acid synthesis, fatty acids and mitochondrial physiology. *Biochim Biophys Acta, 1862*(1), 39-48. doi: 10.1016/j.bbalip.2016.08.011

Kennedy, S. R., Salk, J. J., Schmitt, M. W., & Loeb, L. A. (2013). Ultrasensitive sequencing reveals an age-related increase in somatic mitochondrial mutations that are inconsistent with oxidative damage. [*PLoS Genet, 9*(9), e1003794.

Kim, Y. C., & Guan, K. L. (2015). mTOR: a pharmacologic target for autophagy regulation. *J Clin Invest, 125*(1), 25-32.

Kleff, S., Kemper, B., & Sternglanz, R. (1992). Identification and characterization of yeast mutants and the gene for a cruciform cutting endonuclease. *EMBO J, 11*(2), 699-704.

Kmiec, B., Woloszynska, M., & Janska, H. (2006). Heteroplasmy as a common state of mitochondrial genetic information in plants and animals. *Curr Genet, 50*(3), 149-159.

Kowald, A., Dawson, M., & Kirkwood, T. B. (2014). Mitochondrial mutations and ageing: can mitochondrial deletion mutants accumulate via a size based replication advantage? *J Theor Biol, 340*, 111-118.

Kraytsberg, Y., Schwartz, M., Brown, T. A., Ebralidse, K., Kunz, W. S., Clayton, D. A., ... Khrapko, K. (2004). Recombination of human mitochondrial DNA. *Science, 304*(5673), 981.

Ladoukakis, E. D., & Zouros, E. (2001). Direct evidence for homologous recombination in mussel (Mytilus galloprovincialis) mitochondrial DNA. *Mol Biol Evol, 18*(7), 1168-1175.

Lauri, A., Pompilio, G., & Capogrossi, M. C. (2014). The mitochondrial genome in aging and senescence. . *Ageing Res Rev, 18*, 1-15.

Lehtinen, S. K., Hance, N., El Meziane, A., Juhola, M. K., Juhola, K. M., Karhu, R., ... Jacobs, H. T. (2000). Genotypic stability, segregation and selection in heteroplasmic human cell lines containing np 3243 mutant mtDNA. *Genetics, 154*(1), 363-380.

Lipinski, M. M., Zheng, B., Lu, T., Yan, Z., Py, B. F., Ng, A., ... Yuan, J. (2010). Genome-wide analysis reveals mechanisms modulating autophagy in normal brain aging and in Alzheimer's disease. *Proc Natl Acad Sci U S A, 107*(32), 14164-14169.

Lombes, A., Aure, K., Bellanne-Chantelot, C., Gilleron, M., & Jardel, C. (2014). Unsolved issues related to human mitochondrial diseases. *Biochimie, 100*, 171-176.

McFarland, R., Clark, K. M., Morris, A. A., Taylor, R. W., Macphail, S., Lightowlers, R. N., & Turnbull, D. M. (2002). Multiple neonatal deaths due to a homoplasmic mitochondrial DNA mutation. *Nat Genet, 30*(2), 145-146.

Minczuk, M., Papworth, M. A., Kolasinska, P., Murphy, M. P., & Klug, A. (2006). Sequence-specific modification of mitochondrial DNA using a chimeric zinc finger methylase. [Research Support, Non-U.S. Gov't]. *Proc Natl Acad Sci U S A, 103*(52), 19689-19694.

Mingozzi, F., & High, K. A. (2011). Therapeutic in vivo gene transfer for genetic disease using AAV: progress and challenges. *Nat Rev Genet, 12*(5), 341-355.

Morgan, J. A., Macbeth, M., Broderick, D., Whatmore, P., Street, R., Welch, D. J., & Ovenden, J. R. (2013). Hybridisation, paternal leakage and mitochondrial DNA linearization in three anomalous fish (Scombridae). [*Mitochondrion, 13*(6), 852-861.

Moscou, M. J., & Bogdanove, A. J. (2009). A simple cipher governs DNA recognition by TAL effectors. *Science, 326*(5959), 1501.

Nachman, M. W., Brown, W. M., Stoneking, M., & Aquadro, C. F. (1996). Nonneutral mitochondrial DNA variation in humans and chimpanzees. *Genetics, 142*(3), 953-963.

Narendra, D., Tanaka, A., Suen, D.-F., & Youle, R. J. (2008). Parkin is recruited selectively to impaired mitochondria and promotes their autophagy.. *The Journal of Cell Biology, 183*(5), 795-803.

Nickel, A., Kohlhaas, M., & Maack, C. (2014). Mitochondrial reactive oxygen species production and elimination. *J Mol Cell Cardiol, 73*, 26-33.

Papworth, M., Kolasinska, P., & Minczuk, M. (2006). Designer zinc-finger proteins and their applications. *Gene, 366*(1), 27-38.

Papworth, M., Moore, M., Isalan, M., Minczuk, M., Choo, Y., & Klug, A. (2003). Inhibition of herpes simplex virus 1 gene expression by designer zinc-finger transcription factors. *Proc Natl Acad Sci U S A, 100*(4), 1621-1626.

Payne, B. A., Wilson, I. J., Hateley, C. A., Horvath, R., Santibanez-Koref, M., Samuels, D. C., ... Chinnery, P. F. (2011). Mitochondrial aging is accelerated by anti-retroviral therapy through the clonal expansion of mtDNA mutations.*Nat Genet, 43*(8), 806-810.

Pickrell, A. M., & Youle, R. J. (2015). The roles of PINK1, parkin, and mitochondrial fidelity in Parkinson's disease. *Neuron, 85*(2), 257-273.

Piganeau, G., Gardner, M., & Eyre-Walker, A. (2004). A broad survey of recombination in animal mitochondria. *Mol Biol Evol, 21*(12), 2319-2325.

Poulton, J., Deadman, M. E., Bindoff, L., Morten, K., Land, J., & Brown, G. (1993). Families of mtDNA re-arrangements can be detected in patients with mtDNA deletions: duplications may be a transient intermediate form. [Research Support, Non-U.S. Gov't]. *Hum Mol Genet, 2*(1), 23-30.

Qi, Y., Wei, Y., Wang, Q., Xu, H., Wang, Y., Yao, A., ... Zhou, F. (2016). Heteroplasmy of mutant mitochondrial DNA A10398G and analysis of its prognostic value in non-small cell lung cancer. *Oncol Lett, 12*(5), 3081-3088.

Raap, A. K., Jahangir Tafrechi, R. S., van de Rijke, F. M., Pyle, A., Wahlby, C., Szuhai, K., ... Janssen, G. M. (2012). Non-random mtDNA segregation patterns indicate a metastable heteroplasmic segregation unit in m.3243A>G cybrid cells. *PloS one, 7*(12), e52080.

Rajasimha, H. K., Chinnery, P. F., & Samuels, D. C. (2008). Selection against pathogenic mtDNA mutations in a stem cell population leads to the loss of the 3243A-->G mutation in blood. *Am J Hum Genet, 82*(2), 333-343.

Reddy, P., Ocampo, A., Suzuki, K., Luo, J., Bacman, S. R., Williams, S. L., ... Izpisua Belmonte, J. C. (2015). Selective elimination of mitochondrial mutations in the germline by genome editing. *Cell, 161*(3), 459-469.

Rouzier, C., Bannwarth, S., Chaussenot, A., Chevrollier, A., Verschueren, A., Bonello-Palot, N., ... Paquis-Flucklinger, V. (2012). The MFN2 gene is responsible for mitochondrial DNA instability and optic atrophy 'plus' phenotype. [Research Support, Non-U.S. Gov't]. *Brain, 135*(Pt 1), 23-34.

Ruiz-Pesini, E., Lott, M. T., Procaccio, V., Poole, J. C., Brandon, M. C., Mishmar, D., ... Wallace, D. C. (2007). An enhanced MITOMAP with a global mtDNA mutational phylogeny. *Nucleic Acids Res, 35*(Database issue), D823-828.

Schon, E. A., Rizzuto, R., Moraes, C. T., Nakase, H., Zeviani, M., & DiMauro, S. (1989). A direct repeat is a hotspot for large-scale deletion of human mitochondrial DNA.. *Science, 244*(4902), 346-349.

Schwartz, M., & Vissing, J. (2002). Paternal inheritance of mitochondrial DNA. *N Engl J Med, 347*(8), 576-580.

Schwartz, R. M., & Dayhoff, M. O. (1978). Origins of prokaryotes, eukaryotes, mitochondria, and chloroplasts. *Science, 199*(4327), 395-403.

Sembongi, H., Di Re, M., Bokori-Brown, M., & Holt, I. J. (2007). The yeast Holliday junction resolvase, CCE1, can restore wild-type mitochondrial DNA to human cells carrying rearranged mitochondrial DNA. *Hum Mol Genet, 16*(19), 2306-2314.

Solignac, M., Monnerot, M., & Mounolou, J. C. (1983). Mitochondrial DNA heteroplasmy in Drosophila mauritiana. *Proc Natl Acad Sci U S A, 80*(22), 6942-6946.

Sondheimer, N., Glatz, C. E., Tirone, J. E., Deardorff, M. A., Krieger, A. M., & Hakonarson, H. (2011). Neutral mitochondrial heteroplasmy and the influence of aging. *Hum Mol Genet, 20*(8), 1653-1659.

Srivastava, S., & Moraes, C. T. (2001). Manipulating mitochondrial DNA heteroplasmy by a mitochondrially targeted restriction endonuclease. *Hum Mol Genet, 10*(26), 3093-3099.

Stewart, J. B., & Larsson, N. G. (2014). Keeping mtDNA in shape between generations.*PLoS Genet, 10*(10), e1004670.

Suen, D. F., Narendra, D. P., Tanaka, A., Manfredi, G., & Youle, R. J. (2010). Parkin overexpression selects against a deleterious mtDNA mutation in heteroplasmic cybrid cells. *Proc Natl Acad Sci U S A, 107*(26), 11835-11840.

Tanaka, M., Borgeld, H. J., Zhang, J., Muramatsu, S., Gong, J. S., Yoneda, M., ... Yagi, K. (2002). Gene therapy for mitochondrial disease by delivering restriction endonuclease SmaI into mitochondria. [Research Support, Non-U.S. Gov't]. *J Biomed Sci, 9*(6 Pt 1), 534-541.

Thorburn, D. R., & Dahl, H. H. (2001). Mitochondrial disorders: genetics, counseling, prenatal diagnosis and reproductive options. *Am J Med Genet, 106*(1), 102-114.

Thyagarajan, B., Padua, R. A., & Campbell, C. (1996). Mammalian mitochondria possess homologous DNA recombination activity. *J Biol Chem, 271*(44), 27536-27543.

Villanueva Paz, M., Cotan, D., Garrido-Maraver, J., Cordero, M. D., Oropesa-Avila, M., de La Mata, M., ... Sanchez-Alcazar, J. A. (2016). Targeting autophagy and mitophagy for mitochondrial diseases treatment. *Expert Opin Ther Targets, 20*(4), 487-500.

Wang, D., Kreutzer, D. A., & Essigmann, J. M. (1998). Mutagenicity and repair of oxidative DNA damage: insights from studies using defined lesions. [Review]. *Mutat Res, 400*(1-2), 99-115.

Watanabe, T., Ochiai, H., Sakuma, T., Horch, H. W., Hamaguchi, N., Nakamura, T., ... Mito, T. (2012). Non-transgenic genome modifications in a hemimetabolous insect using zinc-finger and TAL effector nucleases. *Nat Commun, 3*, 1017.

Wei, H., Liu, L., & Chen, Q. (2015). Selective removal of mitochondria via mitophagy: distinct pathways for different mitochondrial stresses. *Biochim Biophys Acta, 1853*(10 Pt B), 2784-2790.

Wolff, J. N., & Gemmell, N. J. (2008). Lost in the zygote: the dilution of paternal mtDNA upon fertilization. *Heredity (Edinb), 101*(5), 429-434.

Ye, K., Lu, J., Ma, F., Keinan, A., & Gu, Z. (2014). Extensive pathogenicity of mitochondrial heteroplasmy in healthy human individuals. *Proc Natl Acad Sci U S A, 111*(29), 10654-10659.

Youle, R. J., & Narendra, D. P. (2011). Mechanisms of mitophagy. [Review]. *Nat Rev Mol Cell Biol, 12*(1), 9-14.

Zimorski, V., Ku, C., Martin, W. F., & Gould, S. B. (2014). Endosymbiotic theory for organelle origins. [Review]. *Curr Opin Microbiol, 22*, 38-48. doi: 10.1016/j.mib.2014.09.008.

Zsurka, G., Kraytsberg, Y., Kudina, T., Kornblum, C., Elger, C. E., Khrapko, K., & Kunz, W. S. (2005). Recombination of mitochondrial DNA in skeletal muscle of individuals with multiple mitochondrial DNA heteroplasmy. *Nat Genet, 37*(8), 873-877.

BIOGRAPHICAL SKETCH

José A. Sánchez Alcázar

Affiliation: Universidad Pablo de Olavide

Education:
B.S. in Biology
Doctor of Medicine, M.D.
PhD in Biochemistry
Residency in Clinical Chemistry
Business Address:
Carretera de Utrera Km 1
Sevilla 41013, Spain

Research and Professional Experience:

Coenzyme Q_{10}, Apoptosis, Mitochondrial diseases

Professional Appointments:

1987-1992	Res. Medical Doctor (Clin. Biochem)	Hospital 12 de Octubre (Madrid), Spain
1993-1995	Posdoctoral Fellow	Fondo de Investigación Sanitaria, Spain.
1996-1997	Posdoctoral Fellow	Schering-Plough
1997-1998	Posdoctoral Fellow	Health Research, Inc. Albany, NY, USA
1998-2000	Posdoctoral Fellow	Spanish Government
2000-2001	Posdoctoral Fellow	Nottingham University, UK
2001-2008	Associate professor	Universidad Pablo de Olavide, Sevilla, Spain
2008-present	Tenured professor	Universidad Pablo de Olavide, Sevilla, Spain

Publications from the Last 3 Years:

López-Escobar B, Cano DA, Rojas A, de Felipe B, Palma F, Sánchez-Alcázar JA, Henderson D, Ybot-González P. The effect of maternal diabetes on the Wnt-PCP pathway during embryogenesis as reflected in the developing mouse eye. López-Escobar B, Cano DA, Rojas A, de Felipe B, Palma F, Sánchez-Alcázar JA, Henderson D, Ybot-González P. *Dis Model Mech.* 2015 Feb;8(2):157-68.

Sánchez-Domínguez B, Bullón P, Román-Malo L, Marín-Aguilar F, Alcocer-Gómez E, Carrión AM, Sánchez-Alcazar JA, Cordero MD. Oxidative stress, mitochondrial dysfunction and, inflammation common events in skin of patients with Fibromyalgia. *Mitochondrion.* 2015;21:69-75.

Alcocer-Gómez E, Garrido-Maraver J, Bullón P, Marín-Aguilar F, Cotán D, Carrión AM, Alvarez-Suarez JM, Giampieri F, Sánchez-Alcazar JA, Battino M, Cordero MD. Metformin and caloric restriction induce an AMPK-dependent restoration of mitochondrial dysfunction in fibroblasts from Fibromyalgia patients. *Biochim Biophys Acta*, 2015, 1852(7):1257-1267.

David Cotán, Marina Villanueva Paz, Elizabet Alcocer-Gómez, Juan Garrido-Maraver1, Manuel Oropesa-Ávila, Mario de la Mata, Ana Delgado Pavón, Isabel de Lavera, Fernando Galán, Patricia Ybot-González, and José A. Sánchez-Alcázar. *AMPK as a target in rare diseases Current Drug Targets*, 2016;17(8):921-31.

Mario de la Mata, David Cotán, Manuel Oropesa-Ávila, Juan Garrido-Maraver, Mario D. Cordero, Marina Villanueva Paz, Ana Delgado Pavón, Elizabet Alcocer-Gómez, Isabel de Lavera, Patricia Ybot-González, Ana Paula Zaderenko, Carmen Ortiz Mellet, José M. García Fernández, José A. Sánchez-Alcázar. Pharmacological Chaperones and Coenzyme Q10 Treatment Improves Mutant β−Glucocerebrosidase Activity and Mitochondrial Function in Neuronopathic Forms of Gaucher Disease. *Scientific Reports*, 2015, 5:10903.

Guillermo López-Lluch, Juan Carlos Rodríguez-Aguilera, Carlos Santos-Ocaña, José Antonio Sánchez-Alcázar, Daniel José Moreno Fernández-Ayala, Claudio Asencio-Salcedo and Plácido Navas. Mitochondrial responsibility in aging process: inocent, suspect or guilty. *Biogerontology* 2015, 16(5):599-620.

Pedro Bullón, Angel M. Carrión, Elísabet Alcocer-Gómez, Juan Garrido-Maraver, Fabiola Marín-Aguilar, Lourdes Román-Malo, Jesus Ruiz-Cabello, Ognjen Culic, Bernhard Ryffel, Lionel Apetoh, François Ghiringhelli, Maurizio Battino, José Antonio Sánchez-Alcazar, Mario D. Cordero. AMPK phosphorylation modulates pain by activation of NLRP3-inflammasome. *Antioxid Redox Signal* 2016, Jan 20;24(3):157-70.

Elisabet Alcocer-Gómez, Cristina Ulecia-Morón, Fabiola Marín-Aguilar · Tatyana Rybkina, Nieves Casas-Barquero, Jesús Ruiz-Cabello, Bernhard Ryffel, Lionel Apetoh, François Ghiringhelli, Pedro Bullón,

José Antonio Sánchez-Alcazar, Angel M. Carrión, Mario D. Cordero. Stress-induced depressive behaviors require a functional NLRP3-inflammasome. *Molecular Neurobiology* 2016, Sep;53(7):4874-82.

Fernando Galán, Isabel de Lavera, David Cotán and José A Sánchez-Alcázar. Mitochondrial myopathy in follow up a patient with chronic fatigue syndrome. *Journal of Investigative Medicine High Impact Case Reports* 2015 Sep 24;3(3):2324709615607908.

Juan Garrido-Maraver; Marina Villanueva Paz; Mario D. Cordero; Juan Bautista-Lorite; Manuel Oropesa-Ávila; Mario de la Mata; Ana Delgado Pavón; Isabel de Lavera; Elizabet Alcocer-Gómez; Fernando Galán; Patricia Ybot González; David Cotán; Sandra Jackson; José A. Sánchez-Alcázar. Critical role of AMP-activated protein kinase in the balance between mitophagy and mitochondrial biogenesis in MELAS disease. *BBA- Molecular Basis of Disease* 2015, 1852(11):2535-53.

Emerging roles of apoptotic microtubules during the execution phase of apoptosis. Manuel Oropesa Ávila; Alejandro Fernández Vega; Juan Garrido Maraver, Marina Villanueva Paz; Isabel De Lavera; Mario De La Mata; Mario D. Cordero; Elizabet Alcocer Gómez; Ana Delgado Pavón; Mónica Álvarez Córdoba; David Cotán; José Antonio Sánchez-Alcázar. *Cytoskeleton* 2015 72(9):435-46.

Marina Villanueva Paz; David Cotán; Mario D. Cordero; Juan Garrido Maraver; Manuel Oropesa-Ávila; Mario de la Mata; Ana Delgado Pavón; Elisabet Alcócer Gómez; Isabel de Lavera; José A. Sánchez Alcázar. Targeting autophagy and mitophagy in mitochondrial diseases treatment. *Expert Opinion on Therapeutic Targets* 2016; 20(4):487-500.

Mario D. Cordero, Elísabet Alcocer-Gómez, Fabiola Marín-Aguilar, Tatyana Rybkina, David Cotán, Antonio Pérez-Pulido, José Miguel Alvarez-Suarez, Maurizio Battino, José Antonio Sánchez-Alcazar, Angel M. Carrión, Ognjen Culic, Pedro Bullón. TÍTULO: Mutation in Cytochrome b gene of mitochondrial DNA in a family with Fibromyalgia is associated with NLRP3-Inflammasome activation. *Journal of Medical Genetics* 2016 Feb; 53(2):113-22.

J. R. Aguilera, V. Venegas, J. M. Olivaa, M. J. Sayagués, M. de Miguel, J. A. Sánchez-Alcázar, M. Arévalo-Rodríguez and A. P. Zaderenko.

Targeted multifunctional tannic acid nanoparticles. *RSC Advances* 2016, 6, 7279-7287.

Dan J Klionsky, ..., José Antonio Sánchez-Alcazar, ..., Guidelines for the use and interpretation of assays for monitoring autophagy (3 edition). *Autophagy*, 2016;12(1):1-222.

Lucía Spangenberga, Martín Grañaa, Gonzalo Greifa, Juan M Suarez-Riverob,d, Karina Krysztalc, Alejandra Tapiée, María Boidie, Valeria Fraga, Aída Lemesg, Rosario Gueçaimburúe, Alfredo Cerisolah, José A Sánchez-Alcázar, Carlos Robelloa, Victor Raggio, Hugo Naya. 3697G>A in MT-ND1 is a causative mutation in mitochondrial diseases. *Mitochondrion* 2016, 28:54-9.

Isabel de Lavera, Ana Delgado Pavón, Marina Villanueva Paz, Manuel Oropesa-Ávila, Mario de la Mata, Elizabet Alcocer-Gómez, Juan Garrido-Maraver, David Cotán, Mónica Álvarez-Córdoba, and José A. Sánchez-Alcázar. The connections among autophagy, inflammasome and mitochondria. *Curr Drug Targets*, 2017, 18, 9.

Marina Villanueva-Paz, Mario D. Cordero, Ana Delgado Pavón, Beatriz Castejón Vega, David Cotán, Mario De la Mata, Manuel Oropesa-Ávila, Elizabet Alcocer-Gomez, Isabel de Lavera, Juan Garrido-Maraver, José Carrascosa, Ana Paula Zaderenko, Jordi Muntané, Manuel de Miguel and José Antonio Sánchez-Alcázar. Amitriptyline induces mitophagy that precedes apoptosis in human HepG2 cells. *Genes & Cancer*, 2016 Jul; 7(7-8):260-277.

Elísabet Alcocer-Gómez, Ognjen Culic, José M. Navarro-Pando, José A. Sánchez-Alcázar, Pedro Bullón. Effect of Coenzyme Q10 in psychopathological symptoms in Fibromyalgia patients. *CNS Neuroscience & Therapeutics* 2017 Feb; 23(2):188-189.

Manuel Oropesa-Ávila, Patricia de la Cruz-Ojeda, Jesús Porcuna, Marina Villanueva-Paz, Alejandro Fernández-Vega, Mario de la Mata, Isabel de Lavera, Juan Miguel Suarez Rivero, Raquel Luzón–Hidalgo, Mónica Álvarez-Córdoba, David Cotán, Ana Paula Zaderenko, Mario D Cordero, and José A. Sánchez-Alcázar. Two coffins and a funeral: early or late caspase activation determines two types of apoptosis induced by DNA damaging agents. *Apoptosis*, 2017, 22(3):421-436.

Juan M. Suárez-Rivero, Marina Villanueva-Paz, Patricia de la Cruz-Ojeda, Mario de la Mata, David Cotán, Manuel Oropesa-Ávila, Isabel de Lavera, Mónica Álvarez-Córdoba, Raquel Luzón-Hidalgo, José A. Sánchez-Alcázar. Mitochondrial dynamics in mitochondrial diseases. *Diseases* 2017, 5, 1.

Mario de la Mata, David Cotán, Manuel Oropesa-Ávila, Marina Villanueva-Paz, Isabel de Lavera, Mónica Álvarez-Córdoba, Raquel Luzón-Hidalgo, Juan M Suárez-Rivero, Gustavo Tiscornia, José A. Sánchez-Alcázar. Coenzyme Q10 partially restores pathological alterations in a macrophage model of Gaucher disease. *Orphan Journal Rare of Diseases*, 2017, 12(1):23.

Tamara Ortiz; Eduardo Díaz-Parrado.; Matilde Illanes.; Ana Fernández-Rodríguez; José Antonio Sánchez-Alcázar; Manuel de Miguel. Amitriptyline down-regulates coenzyme Q10 biosynthesis in lung cancer cells. *European Journal of Pharmacology*, 2017, 797:75-82 .

M. Isabel García-Moreno, Mario de la Mata, Elena M. Sánchez-Fernández, Juan M. Benito, Anotonio Díaz-Quintana, Santos Fustero, Eiji Nanba, Katsumi Higaki, José A. Sánchez-Alcázar, José M. García Fernández, Carmen Ortiz Mellet. Fluorinated Chaperone—β-Cyclodextrin Formulations for β–Glucocerebrosidase Activity Enhancement in Neuronopathic Gaucher Disease. *Journal of Medicinal Chemistry*, 2017, 60(5):1829-1842.

Elísabet Alcocer-Gómez, Nieves Casas-Barquero, Matthew R. Williams, Samuel L.Romero-Guillena, Diego Cañadas-Lozano, Pedro Bullón, José Antonio Sánchez-Alcázar, José M Navarro-Pando, Mario D. Cordero.Differential effect of antidepressant treatment in the inhibition of NLRP3-inflammasome in Major depressive disorder. *Pharmacological research* 2017, 121:114-121.

In: Advances in Health and Disease
Editor: Lowell T. Duncan

ISBN: 978-1-53613-020-1
© 2018 Nova Science Publishers, Inc.

Chapter 4

THE ATTACHMENT AND ITS ROLE IN MEDICAL CARE

Carlo Lai[1],*, Gaia Romana Pellicano[1], Daniela Altavilla[1], Laura Pierro[1], Erika Fazzari[1], Edvaldo Begotaraj[1], Giada Lucarelli[1], Paola Aceto[2] and Massimiliano Luciani[3]

[1]Department of Dynamic and Clinical Psychology
Sapienza University of Rome, Italy
[2]Department of Anesthesiology and Intensive Care,
Gemelli University Hospital, Rome, Italy
[3]Department of Neuroscience Catholic University of
Sacred Heart, Rome, Italy

ABSTRACT

Attachment styles are relational models that lead an individual to seek proximity to a safe or powerful person when threatened. As suggested by attachment theory, the quality of early interpersonal experiences shapes the self-regulate ability during the entire life span and modulate the complex

---

* Corresponding Author E-mail: carlo.lai@uniroma1.it.

relationship between social, cognitive, and emotional variables. The attachment system seems to be strongly involved in the health-related events, due to its self-regulation function. Individuals with physical illness are forced to cope with new people, contexts and experiences that are potential stressors of attachment system. Relational models, thus, seem to have a significant role in health-related psychological processes, in particular, on patients' ability to engage in a fruitful alliance with their physicians. Major chronic conditions and their complex management could broadly take advantage from a safely and trustful relationship between patient and physician. Patient medical adherence is a basic statement in health care and recent studies reported that it is closely associated with the affective relationship between patient and practitioner. Investigating the patient attachment style as a moderator of this relationship could promote clinical interventions aimed to enhance the adherence to medical care, improving health-care outcomes and patient quality of life.

Keywords: medical care, attachment system, diabetes, adherence

1. INTRODUCTION

Attachment is a psychological dimension that explains the "deep and enduring emotional bond that connects one person to another across time and space," (Bowlby, 1969; Ainsworth, 1973). It is characterized by specific behaviors in children, such as "seeking proximity with the attachment figure when upset or threatened" (Bowlby, 1969). According to Bowlby, human attachment originated from an evolutionary strategy that aimed to protect and promote infant survival (Tryphonopoulos et al., 2014). As reported by Vrticka and colleagues (2008), "the functions of attachment were first related to the regulation of proximity-seeking behavior, with the goal to obtain protection and care from another person" (an attachment figure). The attachment could be defined as "a broad theory of social development that describes the origins of the patterns of close interpersonal relationships, interpersonal actions intended to increase an individual's sense of security, particularly in times of stress and needs" (Ravitz et al., 2009).

The attachment theory has its own origin in the classical psychoanalysis, since Bowlby's psychodynamic background. However, the attachment theory largely explains the nature of the first emotional and affective relationships established by the infant with other people, especially with its principal caregiver.

Bowlby's intuitions about the attachment were influenced by the ethology and ecology. Most part of the rationale of this theory came out by the observations he made during his work with disadvantaged children, focusing on the loss and separation (Bowlby, 1944). Meanwhile, the attachment theory has been also influenced by more classic psychological approaches, in particular by M. Klein's object relations theory (1946), by W. Fairbairn's internalized objects (1952) and by Maslow's hierarchy of human's needs (1943).

1.1. Theoretical Basis

Paraphrasing Bowlby, "the attachment can be already observed in the first year of the child's life and becomes mature within this first year" (1969). The attachment theory is a psychological construct which is activated independently, and at the same time, directly and indirectly from the context. On the other hand, what are the main characteristics of the attachment? Primarily, the child behavior is driven by the motivation to interact with the caregiver, that depends from affection to satisfy his own needs. Successively, influenced by cognitive theories, Bowlby introduced the Internal Working Models (IWM) (1969). These are mental representations constructed from the experience of the early relationships. These models postulate that the child interprets the surrounding relational information and uses this to form cognitive schemes, that subsequently guide the child in its reactions and behaviors. Subsequently, Ainsworth (1968) introduced "the secure base strategy" concept, according to which "children, during their interaction, use the caregiver as their secure base for their needs, protection, stability and exploration of the environment" (1968). The attachment is a psychological construct in continuous development during the human's lifespan (Weiss, 1991) and lasts for the whole lifecycle.

1.2. The Attachment System

Ainsworth defined the attachment as an evident form of behavior or as a specific type of reaction that children use in the interaction with the caregiver. Ainsworth (1970), and subsequently Main (1986), distinguished four attachment styles (see Table 1.1).

Table 1.1. The infant attachment dimensions

Secure Attachment	Children who tend to be frightened when are distant from their mother, looking for her, avoiding any other activity they were doing till that moment. After the mother comes back, they continue their playing naturally.
Anxious-Resistant/ Ambivalent Insecure Attachment	Children who tend to be very anxious to the separation and when the mother comes back, is difficult to accept and to be calm. They like to be controlling about their relationship with the mother, but at the same time looking intensively for the caregiver to be attached.
Avoidant Insecure Attachment	Children who tend to develop a relation with the mother not based on reciprocal faithfulness. They are not frightened when mother goes away and shows no reaction when she comes back. Shows no empathy and are not collaborative.
Disorganized/ Disoriented Attachment	Children difficult to be predicted, altering close intimacy with distant relationship with the caregiver. They tend to absorb the mother's preoccupation, showing themselves angry and frightened. They have strange behaviours, rigid and unbelievers about the caregiver's purposes.

Successive studies reported interesting results also about the attachment styles in adulthood (Weiss, 1982; Main et al., 1985; Bretherton et al., 1990).

In adulthood, the attachment is defined as "the stable tendency of an individual to make substantial efforts to seek and maintain proximity to and contact with one or few specific individuals who provide the subjective potential for physical and/or psychological safety and security" (Sperling & Berman, 1994). Some researchers have proposed different categories for the adult attachment system (see Table 1.2) (Obegi & Berant, 2010; Main, Kaplan & Kassidy, 1985; Van Ijzendorn, 1995, Hazard & Shaver, 1987).

Table 1.2. The adult attachment dimensions

The Secure Adults	People who tend to act autonomously, good listeners and with optimized internal working models, who can control emotional intimacy, able to communicate their needs and emotions.
The Preoccupied Adults, (Ambivalent Style)	People who tend to be inconsistent and with changes of mood, tend to be communicative but without good results, not comfortable with intimacy, insecure, anxious, emotional, always need to be attached to someone.
The Dismissive Style (Avoidant Adults),	People who tend to be distant, can control themselves but poor emotionally, detached, sceptic and doubter, with the tendency to reject an intimate relationship, preferring to stay alone.
The Fearful Style (Unresolved Adults)	People who tend to harm their own children with the excuse of the education, have no empathy, with trauma memories who bring back previous fears, tend to be antisocial, don't like rules, aggressive and have difficulty to attune the emotional regulation.

Patterns of attachment are stable from the infancy to the adulthood, but during the lifespan, change according with individual's needs (see Table 1.3).

Table 1.3. Patterns of attachment from infancy to adulthood

Attachment	
Infant	Adult
4 styles	4 styles
MOI	MOI
Complementary	Sexual attraction
Directed from caregiver	Equal age
Secure base effect	Interchangeability of roles
Search for proximity	Bidirectional
Protection	Protection
Separation-anxiety	Separation-anxiety
Exploration	

1.3. Further Contributions

Over recent years, there were other contributions that confirm the relevance of the attachment theory, in particular into clinical psychology (Daniel, 2006). Ravitz et al., (2010) sustained that "adult attachment is becoming increasingly important in psychosomatic research because the attachment influences many biopsychosocial phenomena, including social functioning, coping, stress response, psychological well-being, health behavior and mortality." According to Daniel (2006) "adult attachment patterns are thought to be relatively stable, because new experiences are assimilated to the existing working model, and because the patterns give rise to self-perpetuating interactional behaviors." Moreover, another study confirmed the importance to investigate the adult attachment in the clinical contexts (Maunder & Hunter, 2009). According to their suggestions, prototypic descriptions of patterns of adult attachment may guide clinicians in appreciating individual differences in interpersonal style that affect patients' health (2009). This chapter will be focused, in particular, on the role of the attachment system as a mediator factor between adherence and medical care in chronic disease.

2. Attachment and Medical Care

The attachment theory provides an interesting framework for the comprehension of health-related issues. The attachment bonding aims to provide support and care; however, when an illness is the threat, rarely the familiar others can offer safety because they do not often have the expertise to manage illness (Salmon & Young, 2009). Several studies investigated the attachment theory in clinical relationships because, during an illness, the practitioner becomes whom as having the expertise and power to provide safety (Wright et al., 2004; Salander, 2002; Tan et al., 2005; Ciechanowski 2002).

Into the field of the health, the attachment theory acquires an important role as a factor that could affect the relationship between patients and public health care, and, consequently, on the treatment outcomes.

A collaborative patient-provider relationship may be particularly important and is one of the most significant determinants that has a positive influence on the outcomes of an optimal treatment.

As reported by the Committee on Quality of Health Care in America (2001), a patient-centered care that emphasizes the empathy and responsiveness to patients' needs, values and preferences increase patient's participation and autonomy. However, the relationship between patient and provider is, by definition, an asymmetric relationship. Promoting patients as equal partners enhances respect for their autonomy and rights, nevertheless, people who are seriously ill want less involvement in care decisions (Degner & Sloan, 1992). Moreover, patients mostly seek health care because they are sick, or because they fear illness, and want practitioners to help them (Say, 2006), looking at themselves as vulnerable and dependent and at the practitioner as expert and caring (Callahan, 2001). There is a diversity in the way in which patients prefer to interact with clinicians, ranging from patients who prefer few contacts with the physician to those requesting more close and confidential relationships.

Understanding the factors that affect these variations in patient interaction styles and the patients' engagement modality with clinicians may be very important to propose effective health cares (Lai et al., 2016b; Aceto et al., 2016; Tonioni et al., 2012).

Considering that the patients seek a relationship with practitioners when they are afraid and vulnerable, in order to feel themselves safer, the attachment theory (Bowlby, 1969) represents a well suited psychological framework that may deepen the patient-health care relationship. Naturally, the attachment bonding aims to seek and give comfort and proximity, and the main interest is in feelings: "it is a theory about feeling safe rather than being safe" (Salmon & Young, 2009). As suggested by attachment theory, the quality of people's early interpersonal experiences shapes their ability to self-regulate during their entire life span, developing 'mental models' of oneself and others mental and behavioral functioning (Peleg et al., 2016; Salmon & Young, 2009). The regulatory function of attachment style moderates the complex relationship between social, cognitive, and emotional variables (Bodie et al., 2010; Vilchinsky et al., 2015; Mikulincer et al., 2003). Due to its self-regulation function, attachment system has been studied as strongly involved in health-related events, mainly because a diagnosis of illness is a new challenge and the patients should trust in new stranger people, in a new environment and, during an eventual hospitalization, there is also a separation from significant others, and all of which are potential attachment-related stressors (Peleg, et al., 2016; Hunter & Maunder, 2001). Moreover, attachment relationships are classically thought as the result of repeated interactions with the caregiver; however, in clinical settings, the encounters are usually brief and with unfamiliar practitioners who cannot offer 'on demand' proximity. One possible suggestion is that the patients' mental models of self and other help to construct the image of the practitioner and the future interactions with him. Attachment styles, therefore, seem to have a significant role in health-related psychological processes (Pietromonaco et al., 2013; Maunder & Hunter, 2015), since they are in dialectic balance between individuals' autonomy and dependence (Salmon & Young, 2009).

A previous study (Hunter & Maunder, 2001) suggested that individuals with high levels of anxious attachment have little confidence in their ability to cope with own illness by themselves and employ a great amount of means to keep their significant others and their medical team regularly engaged. When facing a threat, highly anxiously attached individuals are more sensitive and responsive to other's opinions and suggestions than people with low anxiety attachment (Peleg et al., 2016). Coherently, Ciechanowski and colleagues (2002) found that people with anxious attachment style tend to use health services more frequently compared to individuals with avoidance attachment style, reporting also more physical symptoms and showing more hopelessness. On the other hand, an avoidant attachment style leads patients to a general unwillingness to seek help (Mikulincer & Shaver, 2007). Highly avoidant individuals are more affected by their own perceptions and less by social feedback than others with low avoidant attachment (Peleg et al., 2016). Moreover, patients with avoidant attachment style are likely to ignore pain signals or appraise them as posing little threat (Meredith et al., 2005) and tend to mistrust the others and perceive as ineffective the medical personnel, because dependence and closeness are detected as stressful (Maunder & Hunter, 2015; 2009). Vilchinsky and colleagues (2015) suggested that, in a poor health situation, avoidant individuals modulate their self-regulation relying on own internal resources, in particular cognitive perceptions of illness.

Therefore, seems that anxiously attached people consider health threats a way to keep others engaged, while avoidant-attached people cope with illness by means of high self-confidence. Secure-attached people are reported as more likely to evaluate events realistically and respond appropriately to stressors such as pain (Mikulincer et al., 1998; Feeney et al., 1996; Simpson et al., 1994), thus obtaining appropriate and timely intervention (Jimenez, 2016).

The way in which patients imagine and consider their own relationship with the health care system and the practitioner has a great impact on the regularity of the clinical visits and on the assumption of the prescribed treatment (Bennett et al., 2011). An irregular treatment and follow-up are associated with worse short- and long-term health outcomes, whereas regular visits contribute to health improvements (Alarcon et al., 2002). A secure attachment style, therefore, represents a significant determinant for successful medical treatment. Recent studies reported the association with patients' secure attachment style and the adherence to the medical treatment (Bennett et al., 2011; Niederhauser, 2001). Adherence is a basic, but rarely met, assumption in health care (DiMatteo et al., 1998), intimately connected to the patient-practitioner relationship and the trust of the patient toward the health care system (DiMatteo, 2004).

2.1. Adherence

Adherence is defined as "the extent of which the patient's behavior matches the prescriber's recommendations" (Horne et al., 2005). It has been adopted as an alternative to the term "compliance" to emphasize that the patient is free to decide to attempt or not the medical recommendations (Horne et al., 2005).

Adherence to the treatment is probably the most daunting challenge today's health professionals have to face up. It can be a source of great concern and frustration. Statistics on non-adherence are alarming: despite the efforts made in recent years to find a solution, 20% to 80% of patients who are supposed to take medication are non-adherent (Brown et al., 2008).

Patients may be non-adherent during different stages of their treatment; they could follow or not the first medical prescription in a single case ("primary adherence") or they could take the dispensed medications as prescribed, during a more prolonged observation period ("secondary adherence") (Hugtenburg et al., 2013; Raebel et al., 2014). Non-adherence, as well as having an impact on the treatment outcome, may also have a significant impact on healthcare costs that may be justified by an increase of requests to hospitalization, laboratory analysis, recourse to first aid services, and increased costs for drugs. (Dragomir et al., 2010; Huang et al., 2017; Lopez-Valcarcel et al., 2017; Pasma et al., 2017; Roebuck et al., 2011; Latremouille-Viau et al., 2017; Dobbels et al., 2017). The reasons why a patient decides not to follow the treatment, or to respect it partially, may be intentional or unintentional (Hugtenburg et al., 2013; Lehane et al., 2007). Intentional non-adherence can be considered as a rational decision-making process in which the patient actively decides to use or not to use the treatment, or to follow the treatment recommendations. Unintentional non-adherence refers to unplanned behaviour associated with the complexity of a medication regimen (not knowing how to use the medicines) and the patient's memory, for example, forgetting to take the medication at the prescribed time and poor recall of the instructions provided by the practitioner (Hugtenburg et al., 2013; Lowry et al., 2005; Bangalore et al., 2007; Lehane et al., 2007).

A study on cardiovascular disease reported that after the onset of a cardiac problem, in a follow-up after 5 years, patients showed a poor adherence to follow-up visits, whereas the adherence to pharmacological care was greater. As consequence, a poor adherence to second-prevention factors increased the probability of recurrence and mortality in this type of patients (Salari et al., 2016). Moreover, adherence to medication therapy in post-operative stage could prevent organ rejection (Dobbels et al., 2017).

Poor adherence may be influenced by several factors, such as the patient's belief, a lack of trust in the therapy or in the practitioner, contextual factors (e.g., social support and socio-economic status), and/or an insufficient communication between patient and provider (Hugtenburg et al., 2013; Ingersoll et al., 2008; Clifford et al., 2007; Bangalore et al., 2007; van Dulmen et al., 2007). Non-adherence was influenced by psychological variables especially when the therapeutic regimen is complex and required high costs (Aceto et al., 2015; Hugtenburg et al., 2013; van Dijk et al., 2007; Steiner, 2012; Bryson et al., 2008; Hicks et al., 2007). Calip and colleagues (2017) reported that the presence of anxiety, depression and post-traumatic stress disorder is related to a greater probability of non-adherence in the cases of complex treatment (Calip et al., 2017). Findings of recent studies on patients affected by chronic kidney disease showed an association between psychological factors and difficulties to adhere to the treatment and to the dietetic regimen (Lai et al., 2017a; 2015; 2014).

Chronic disease implies a long – term use of pharmacotherapy, thus a high level of adherence to medical prescriptions. Studies suggest that 50% of patients on long-term therapy are non-adherent after one year. It makes patients at risk to severely compromise treatment outcomes and increasing mortality (Brown et al., 2008).

3. ATTACHMENT STYLE, CHRONIC DISEASES AND ADHERENCE

Chronic disease is defined as a disease "long in duration—often with a long latency period and protracted clinical course; of multi-factorial etiology; with no definite cure; gradual changes over time, asynchronous evolution and heterogeneity in population susceptibility" (Bentzen et al., 2003; Martin et al., 2007). The World Health Organization identifies the chronic diseases in cardiovascular diseases, stroke, cancer, chronic respiratory diseases and diabetes; these are the leading cause of mortality in the world, representing 60% of all deaths (WHO, 2017). Also asthma, digestive diseases, neurologic disorders, mental and behavioural disorders, kidney diseases, gynecologic disorders, hemoglobinopathies, musculoskeletal disorders, congenital anomalies, skin, sense-organ, and oral disorders are defined as chronic diseases associated with lower percentage (19.6%) of deaths in 2010, compared to the main types of chronic disease previously cited, and an accounted 54.8% of disability-adjusted life-years (DALYs), known as the sum of years of life lost from premature death and years lived with disability (Murray et al., 2013). All of these diseases are also known as non-communicable diseases (NCDs) (Hunter et al., 2013) because these "are not passed from person to person and are of long duration and generally slow progression" (WHO, 2017).

The relational dimension has a critical role in the management of chronic disease. Several studies showed that a positive relationship between the clinician and patient, is associated with adherence, satisfaction with care, and favourable treatment response (Paone et al., 2017; Thompson et al., 2003; Di Blasi et al., 2001; Kaplan et al., 1989). Patients in such a relationship may experience better-perceived health and less distress and impairment (Jackson et al., 2001).

When dealing with medical care, attachment systems that emphasize discomfort communication, seeking help, trusting and personal vulnerability, are inevitably involved. An organized biological system that responds to the perception of the dangers of survival by approaching a protective figure is triggered by illness when is experienced pain, disability, loss or separation from loved ones and is obliged to lean on clinician's care who are relatively foreigners (De Cosmo, et al., 2008).

Several studies, in different chronic disease, show as attachment systems have an influence on the adherence and consequently on the outcomes.

3.1. Diabetes

Diabetes is a common chronic disease that is associated with considerable morbidity and mortality: individuals with diabetes are at greater risk of long-term complications such as kidney disease, peripheral vascular disease, lower extremity ulcers and amputations, retinopathy, and neuropathy.

Prevalence of diabetes in adults worldwide is estimated to be 4.0% in 1995 and to rise to 5.4% by the year 2025. It is higher in developed than in developing countries. The number of adults with diabetes in the world will rise from 135 million in 1995 to 300 million in the year 2025 (King et al., 1995).

A cause of diabetic complications and higher costs is the inadequate glycemic control: proper management of diabetes can delay complications, reduce mortality, and reduce the costs of diabetes care (García-Pérez et al., 2013). Research has shown that aggressive glycemic control can reduce long-term complications in patients with type 1 or type 2 diabetes and result in considerable medical cost savings.

Ciechanowski and colleagues (2004) demonstrated that attachment style was associated with a higher risk for poor glycemic control. Researchers hypothesized that patients who were more self-reliant and less trusting of others might have poorer collaboration with health care providers, which might adversely affect diabetes self-care. Patients with a dismissing attachment style were less adherent with diet, exercise, foot care, and oral hypoglycemic medications were more likely to smoke, and viewed the patient-provider relationship less favorably as compared with patients with a secure attachment style.

The relationship between dismissing attachment style and adherence with self-care was mediated through the patient-provider relationship: this has relevance from a population-based perspective because 25% of the general population has a dismissing attachment style.

The findings in diabetes' studies are consistent with characteristics of dismissing attachment style. People with this style may be more likely to find social interactions unrewarding and to view others as consistently unavailable or incapable of providing care and thus may tend to avoid relying on others. Dismissing attached individuals may show themselves to health care providers as invulnerable and not in need of provider's care or expertise. They may not elaborate on their problems, symptoms, illness, or the effect of their illness because of reluctance to elicit support from others.

3.2. Cancer

Social support is associated with a decrease in psychological symptoms and a better quality of life in cancer patients (Lai et al., 2017; 2016b). Yilmaz Ozpolat and colleagues (2014), in a study, have investigated the role of attachment dimensions on social and psychological adjustment to cancer and have explored the social and psychological adjustments, and medical adherence, among patients with cancer.

The results of their study showed that an avoidant attachment style was related to difficulties in social relationships and an increase in psychological distress following a cancer diagnosis. People who perceive more social support orient to health care more easily than people who perceive less social availability. It was shown that a higher level of perceived social support has a positive impact in adjustment to family relationships and leads to experiencing less psychological distress than in people who perceived less social support. Considering the complicated nature of cancer, a multi-perspective approach should be applied during the treatment process, and it is important to determine the psychosocial factors and the causal pathways by which they lead to a better adjustment, in developing effective interventions.

3.3. Inflammatory Bowel Diseases

Inflammatory bowel diseases (IBD) are chronic disorders affecting psychological well-being, quality of life, social interactions, and close interpersonal relationships of patients affected.

In a recent study, Agostini and colleagues (2014) compared the attachment dimensions between IBD patients and healthy controls evaluating the impact of these dimensions on the quality of life in IBD patients. The results showed that in IBD patients the close interpersonal relationships were characterized by an insecure attachment that, in turn, was a significant predictor of quality of life. This finding suggests plausible insights for psychological interventions in IBD patients with poor quality of life.

3.4. Arthritis

Arthritis is one of the most common chronic pain conditions and a major source of disability worldwide (Arthritis Society, 2010) that can take many different forms: joint pain, inflammation, and functional limitations. Arthritis' symptoms, creating stress and difficulties in management daily activities, can have a negative impact on quality of life. Coping with stressors of the arthritis is a challenge for the individual who suffers from this illness.

Sirois and Gick (2016) evaluated how insecure attachment was linked to arthritis adjustment in a sample of 365 people with arthritis. The results showed indirect and direct associations of anxious and avoidant attachment with greater appraisals of disease-related threat, less perceived social support, and less coping efficacy. There was evidence of reappraisal processes for avoidant but not anxious attachment. These findings highlight the importance of considering attachment style when assessing how people cope with the daily challenges of arthritis.

3.5. Lupus

Systemic lupus erythematosus (SLE) is a prototypical autoimmune disease with a diverse array of clinical manifestations characterized by the presence of anti-nuclear autoantibodies produced by uncontrolled over-activated B cells (Zhan, Guo, Lu, 2016).

In an interesting study, Barbosa and colleagues have investigated attachment style, personality, psychopathological morbidity and quality of life in patients affected by lupus comparing with a healthy volunteer group. The results of the study have shown that SLE patients adopted, mostly, an anxious, insecure attachment style. Moreover, they have found statistically significant and positive correlations between the insecure attachment styles and psychopathological morbidity, they also have noticed negative associations with the dimensions of quality of life. Since SLE has specific and particular characteristics that lead to insecure attachment styles, psychopathological morbidity and impairment, specifics and complementary psychotherapeutic interventions are need.

3.6. Kidney Disease

Chronic kidney disease (CKD) is a highly prevalent condition in the world. Neurological, psychological, and cognitive disorders, related to CKD, could contribute to the morbidity, mortality, and poor quality of life of these patients (Lai et al., 2016c; 2016d).

Chronic kidney disease, also known as a kidney failure, is a slow progressive loss of kidney function over a period of several years. It occurs when kidneys are no longer able to clean toxins and waste product from the blood and perform their functions to full capacity. Renal transplantation represents the end stage of the chronic kidney failure treatment, after a long period of immunosuppressive therapy. Then, it implies strict adherence to the treatment before and after the renal transplantation.

A recent study (Calia et al., 2015) investigated the association between attachment style, compliance, quality of life and renal function in adult patients after kidney transplantation. The results showed that higher levels of insecure attachment (anxious or avoidant) were significantly associated with a worse compliance level and low quality of life. Patients with high levels of avoidant relationship had a low perception of their own mental health and they reported a worse compliance with higher values of creatinine, then lower renal functioning. The results of this study highlight the importance of evaluating the attachment style in adult kidney transplant patients in order to increase their compliance, emphasising the role of attachment style in patient's outcome after renal transplantation. Similarly, Calia et al. (2015a; 2011) showed that insecure attachment style (relationships as secondary and discomfort with closeness) in the mother living donor renal transplant recipients, was significantly associated with worse quality of life (vitality and mental health). It highlights that a more avoidant relationship with the mother can negatively affect the post-transplant outcome.

A recent study (Calia et al., 2015b) showed that the inability to recognize and express emotions, as well as the ability to manage negative emotions, may affect compliance and quality of life of renal transplant patients, highlighting the importance of the emotional regulation, that has its origin in the earlier attachment relationship with the caregivers.

CONCLUSION

At today, the adherence to complex treatment is probably the most daunting challenge that health professionals have to face up. Chronic disease is a disease with long duration and protracted clinical course that implies a long – term use of pharmacotherapy, thus a high level of adherence to medical prescriptions.

Low adherence may be influenced by several factors, such as patient factors, environmental or contextual factors, but the relational dimension seems to have a critical role in the management of chronic disease.

According to Bowlby's attachment theory, the quality of people's early interpersonal experiences shapes their ability to self-regulate during their entire life span, developing 'mental models' of oneself and others mental and behavioral functioning (Peleg et al., 2017; Salmon & Young, 2009). The regulatory function of attachment style moderates the complex relationship between social, cognitive, and emotional variables.

Considering that patients with chronic illness are in a state of fear and vulnerability, Bowlby's attachment theory might make a strong contribution to understanding how they relate to practitioners. In fact, several studies in different chronic disease showed as attachment systems have an influence on the adherence and consequently on the outcomes.

People with avoidant attachment style have a general unwillingness to seek help, they are more affected by their own perceptions and less by social feedback. Moreover, patients with avoidant attachment style tend to mistrust the others and perceive as ineffective the medical personnel, because dependence and closeness are detected as stressful; while, people with anxious attachment style, tend to use health services more frequently compared to individuals with avoidance attachment style, reporting also more physical symptoms and showing more hopelessness.

These different modalities of relating to the clinical professionals and to the care system influence the adherence to the treatment. For this reason, knowing the style of attachment of the patient could inform clinicians how to work with patients who are less engaged in the health care relationship. Moreover, the planning of psychological interventions to support a patient and to mediate the doctor-to-patient relationship could support a greater adherence and more positive outcomes of the treatment in chronic illness, increasing the quality of life of the patient and reducing the care cost.

REFERENCES

Aceto, P., Perilli, V., Lai, C., Ciocchetti, P., Vitale, F., & Sollazzi, L. (2015). Postoperative cognitive dysfunction after liver transplantation. *General hospital psychiatry*, *37*(2), 109-115.

Aceto, P., Lai, C., Perilli, V., Sacco, T., Modesti, C., Raffaelli, M., & Sollazzi, L. (2016). Factors affecting acute pain perception and analgesics consumption in patients undergoing bariatric surgery. *Physiology & behavior*, 163, 1-6.

Agostini, A., Moretti, M., Calabrese, C., Rizzello, F., Gionchetti, P., Ercolani, M., & Campieri, M. (2014). Attachment and quality of life in patients with inflammatory bowel disease. *International journal of colorectal disease, 29*(10), 1291-1296.

Ainsworth, M. D. S. (1969). Object relations, dependency, and attachment: A theoretical review of the infant-mother relationship. *Child development,* 969-1025.

Ainsworth, M. D. S., & Bell, S. M. (1970). Attachment, exploration, and separation: Illustrated by the behavior of one-year-olds in a strange situation. *Child development*, 49-67.

Ainsworth, M. D. S., Bell, S. M., Blehar, M. C., & Main, M. (1971, April). Physical contact: A study of infant responsiveness and its relation to maternal handling. *In biennial meeting of the Society for Research in Child Development*, Minneapolis, MN.

Ainsworth, M. (1973). The Development of Infant-mother Attachment [w:] B. Caldwell, HN Ricciuti (red.), *Review of Child Development Research*, 1–94.

Ainsworth, M. D. S. (1982). *Attachment: Retrospect and prospect*. basic books.

Alarcón, G. S., McGwin, G., Brooks, K., Roseman, J. M., Fessler, B. J., Sanchez, M. L., ... & Reveille, J. D. (2002). Systemic lupus erythematosus in three ethnic groups. XI. Sources of discrepancy in perception of disease activity: a comparison of physician and patient visual analog scale scores. *Arthritis Care & Research*, *47*(4), 408-413.

Baker, A. (2001). Crossing the quality chasm: A new health system for the 21st century. *BMJ: British Medical Journal*, *323*(7322), 1192.

Bangalore, S., Kamalakkannan, G., Parkar, S., & Messerli, F. H. (2007). Fixed-dose combinations improve medication compliance: a meta-analysis. *The American journal of medicine*, *120*(8), 713-719.

Barbosa, F., Ferreira, C., Patrício, P., Mota, C., Alcântara, C., & Barbosa, A. (2010). Attachment style in patients with systemic lupus erythematosus. *Acta Médica Portuguesa*, *23*(1), 51-62.

Bennett, J. K., Fuertes, J. N., Keitel, M., & Phillips, R. (2011). The role of patient attachment and working alliance on patient adherence, satisfaction, and health-related quality of life in lupus treatment. *Patient education and counseling*, *85*(1), 53-59.

Bentzen, N. (Ed.). (2003). *WONCA dictionary of general/family practice*. Wonca International Classification Committee.

Bodie, G. D., Burleson, B. R., Gill-Rosier, J., McCullough, J. D., Holmstrom, A. J., Rack, J. J., et al. (2010). Explaining the impact of attachment style on evaluations of supportive messages: A dual-process framework. *Communication Research, 38*, 228–247.

Bowlby, J. (1944). Forty-four juvenile thieves: their characters and home-life. *The international journal of psycho-analysis, 25*, 107.

Bowlby, J. (1969). *Attachment, Vol. 1 of Attachment and loss.*

Bowlby, J. (2008). *A secure base: Parent-child attachment and healthy human development.* Basic books.

Bretherton, I., Ridgeway, D., & Cassidy, J. (1990). Assessing internal working models of the attachment relationship. *Attachment in the preschool years: Theory, research, and intervention, 273*, 308.

Brown, M. T., & Bussell, J. K. (2011). Medication adherence: WHO cares? *In Mayo Clinic Proceedings, 86*(4), 304-314.

Bryson, C. L., Au, D. H., Sun, H., Williams, E. C., Kivlahan, D. R., & Bradley, K. A. (2008). Alcohol screening scores and medication nonadherence. *Annals of Internal Medicine, 149*(11), 795-803.

Calia, R., Lai, C., Aceto, P., Luciani, M., Camardese, G., Lai, S., ... & Romagnoli, J. (2015). Attachment style predict compliance, quality of life and renal function in adult patients after kidney transplant: preliminary results. *Renal failure, 37*(4), 678-680.

Calia, R., Lai, C., Aceto, P., Pascolo, G., Lai, S., Romagnoli, J., & Citterio, F. (2015a). Emotional management and quality of life in mother living versus multi-organ donor renal transplant recipients. *Journal of health psychology*, 1359105315604378.

Calia, R., Lai, C., Aceto, P., Luciani, M., Camardese, G., Lai, S., ... & Pedroso, J. A. (2015b). Emotional self-efficacy and alexithymia may affect compliance, renal function and quality of life in kidney transplant recipients: Results from a preliminary cross-sectional study. *Physiology & behavior, 142*, 152-154.

Calia, R., Lai, C., Aceto, P., Luciani, M., Saraceni, C., Lai, S., ... & Citterio, F. (2011, May). Preoperative psychological factors predicting graft rejection in patients undergoing kidney transplant: a pilot study. In *Transplantation proceedings* (Vol. 43, No. 4, pp. 1006-1009). Elsevier.

Calip, G. S., Xing, S., Jun, D. H., Lee, W. J., Hoskins, K. F., & Ko, N. Y. (2017). Polypharmacy and Adherence to Adjuvant Endocrine Therapy for Breast Cancer. *Journal of Oncology Practice,* JOP-2016.

Callahan, D. (2001). Our need for caring. *The lost art of caring: a challenge to health professionals, families, communities, and society,* 11-24.

Ciechanowski, P. S., Hirsch, I. B., & Katon, W. J. (2002). Interpersonal predictors of HbA1c in patients with type 1 diabetes. *Diabetes Care, 25*(4), 731-736.

Ciechanowski, P. S., Walker, E. A., Katon, W. J., & Russo, J. E. (2002). Attachment theory: a model for health care utilization and somatization. *Psychosomatic Medicine, 64*(4), 660-667.

Ciechanowski, P., Russo, J., Katon, W., Von Korff, M., Ludman, E., Lin, E., ... & Bush, T. (2004). Influence of patient attachment style on self-care and outcomes in diabetes. *Psychosomatic Medicine, 66*(5), 720-728.

Clifford, S., Barber, N., & Horne, R. (2008). Understanding different beliefs held by adherers, unintentional nonadherers, and intentional nonadherers: application of the necessity–concerns framework. *Journal of psychosomatic research, 64*(1), 41-46.

Coulter, A. (1999). Paternalism or partnership?: Patients have grown up— And there's no going back. *BMJ: British Medical Journal, 319*(7212), 719.

Daniel, S. I. (2006). Adult attachment patterns and individual psychotherapy: A review. *Clinical Psychology Review, 26*(8), 968-984.

De Cosmo, G., Congedo, E., Lai, C., Primieri, P., Dottarelli, A., & Aceto, P. (2008). Preoperative psychologic and demographic predictors of pain perception and tramadol consumption using intravenous patient-controlled analgesia. *The Clinical journal of pain, 24*(5), 399-405.

Degner, L. F., & Sloan, J. A. (1992). Decision making during serious illness: what role do patients really want to play? *Journal of clinical epidemiology, 45*(9), 941-950.

Dewitte, M., & De Houwer, J. (2008). Adult attachment and attention to positive and negative emotional face expressions. *Journal of Research in Personality, 42*(2), 498-505.

Di Blasi, Z., Harkness, E., Ernst, E., Georgiou, A., & Kleijnen, J. (2001). Influence of context effects on health outcomes: a systematic review. *The Lancet, 357*(9258), 757-762.

DiMatteo, M. R. (2004). The role of effective communication with children and their families in fostering adherence to pediatric regimens. *Patient education and counseling, 55*(3), 339-344.

DiMatteo, M. R., & Lepper, H. S. (1998). Promoting adherence to courses of treatment: Mutual collaboration in the physician-patient relationship. *Health communication research: A guide to developments and directions*, 75-86.

Dobbels, F., De Bleser, L., Berben, L., Kristanto, P., Dupont, L., Nevens, F., ... & De Geest, S. (2017). Efficacy of a medication adherence enhancing intervention in transplantation: The maestro-tx trial. *The Journal of Heart and Lung Transplantation*.

Dragomir, A., Côté, R., Roy, L., Blais, L., Lalonde, L., Bérard, A., & Perreault, S. (2010). Impact of adherence to antihypertensive agents on clinical outcomes and hospitalization costs. *Medical care, 48*(5), 418-425.

Fairbairn, W. R. D. (1954). *An object-relations theory of the personality*.

Feeney, B. C., & Kirkpatrick, L. A. (1996). Effects of adult attachment and presence of romantic partners on physiological responses to stress. *Journal of personality and social psychology, 70*(2), 255.

García-Pérez, L. E., Álvarez, M., Dilla, T., Gil-Guillén, V., & Orozco-Beltrán, D. (2013). Adherence to therapies in patients with type 2 diabetes. *Diabetes Therapy, 4*(2), 175-194.

González, L. V. B., Librero, J., García-Sempere, A., Peña, L. M., Bauer, S., Puig-Junoy, J., ... & Sanfélix-Gimeno, G. (2017). Effect of cost sharing on adherence to evidence-based medications in patients with acute coronary syndrome. *Heart (British Cardiac Society)*.

Hazan, C., & Shaver, P. (1987). Romantic love conceptualized as an attachment process. *Journal of personality and social psychology, 52*(3), 511.

Hicks, P. L., Mulvey, K. P., Chander, G., Fleishman, J. A., Josephs, J. S., Korthuis, P. T., ... & HIV Research Network. (2007). The impact of illicit drug use and substance abuse treatment on adherence to HAART. *AIDS care, 19*(9), 1134-1140.

Horne, R., Weinman, J., Barber, N., Elliott, R., Morgan, M., Cribb, A., & Kellar, I. (2005). Concordance, adherence and compliance in medicine taking. *London: NCCSDO, 2005*, 40-6.

Huang, C. Y., Nguyen, P. A. A., Clinciu, D. L., Hsu, C. K., Lu, J. C. R., Yang, H. C., ... & Chang, P. L. (2017). A personalized medication management platform (PMMP) to improve medication adherence: A randomized control trial. *Computer Methods and Programs in Biomedicine, 140*, 275-281.

Hugtenburg, J. G., Timmers, L., Elders, P. J., Vervloet, M., & van Dijk, L. (2013). Definitions, variants, and causes of nonadherence with medication: a challenge for tailored interventions. *Patient Prefer Adherence, 7*, 675-682.

Hulka, B. S., Cassel, J. C., Kupper, L. L., & Burdette, J. A. (1976). Communication, compliance, and concordance between physicians and patients with prescribed medications. *American journal of public health, 66*(9), 847-853.

Hunter, D. J., & Reddy, K. S. (2013). Noncommunicable diseases. *New England Journal of Medicine, 369*(14), 1336-1343.

Hunter, J. J., & Maunder, R. G. (2001). Using attachment theory to understand illness behavior. *General hospital psychiatry, 23*(4), 177-182.

Ingersoll, K. S., & Cohen, J. (2008). The impact of medication regimen factors on adherence to chronic treatment: a review of literature. *Journal of behavioral medicine, 31*(3), 213-224.

Jackson, J. L., Chamberlin, J., & Kroenke, K. (2001). Predictors of patient satisfaction. *Social science & medicine, 52*(4), 609-620.

Jimenez, X. F. (2016). Attachment in medical care: A review of the interpersonal model in chronic disease management. *Chronic illness, 13*(1):14-27.

Kaplan, S. H., Greenfield, S., & Ware Jr, J. E. (1989). Assessing the effects of physician-patient interactions on the outcomes of chronic disease. *Medical care, 27*(3), 110-127.

King, H., Aubert, R. E., & Herman, W. H. (1998). Global burden of diabetes, 1995–2025: prevalence, numerical estimates, and projections. *Diabetes care, 21*(9), 1414-1431.

Klein, M. (1946). Notes on some schizoid mechanisms. *The International journal of psycho-analysis, 27*, 99.

Lai, C., Luciani, M., Galli, F., Morelli, E., Cappelluti, R., Penco, I., ... & Lombardo, L. (2015). Attachment style dimensions can affect prolonged grief risk in caregivers of terminally ill patients with cancer. *American Journal of Hospice and Palliative Medicine, 32*(8), 855-860.

Lai, C., Aceto, P., Luciani, M., Fazzari, E., Cesari, V., Luciano, S., ... & Lai, S. (2016, March). Externally oriented thinking predicts phosphorus levels in dialyzed patients. In *Transplantation proceedings* (Vol. 48, No. 2, pp. 309-310). Elsevier.

Lai, C., Luciani, M., Di Mario, C., Galli, F., Morelli, E., Ginobbi, P., ... & Lombardo, L. (2017). Psychological impairments burden and spirituality in caregivers of terminally ill cancer patients. *European Journal of Cancer Care*.

Lai, C., Borrelli, B., Ciurluini, P., & Aceto, P. (2016b). Sharing information about cancer with one's family is associated with improved quality of life. *Psycho-Oncology*.

Lai, C., Aceto, P., Luciani, M., Fazzari, E., Cesari, V., Luciano, S., ... & Lai, S. (2017a). Emotional management and biological markers of dietetic regimen in chronic kidney disease patients. *Renal failure, 39*(1), 173-178.

Lai, C., Aceto, P., Petrucci, I., Castelnuovo, G., Callari, C., Giustacchini, P., ... & Raffaelli, M. (2016c). The influence of preoperative psychological factors on weight loss after bariatric surgery: A preliminary report. *Journal of health psychology*, 1359105316677750.

Lai, S., Mecarelli, O., Pulitano, P., Romanello, R., Davi, L., Zarabla, A., ... & Mitterhofer, A. P. (2016d). Neurological, psychological, and cognitive disorders in patients with chronic kidney disease on conservative and replacement therapy. *Medicine, 95*(48).

Lai, S., Mariotti, A., Coppola, B., Lai, C., Aceto, P., Dimko, M., ... & Cianci, R. (2014). Uricemia and homocysteinemia: nontraditional risk factors in the early stages of chronic kidney disease—preliminary data. *Eur Rev Med Pharmacol Sci, 18*(7), 1010-1017.

Latremouille-Viau, D., Guerin, A., Gagnon-Sanschagrin, P., Dea, K., Cohen, B. G., & Joseph, G. J. (2017). Health Care Resource Utilization and Costs in Patients with Chronic Myeloid Leukemia with Better Adherence to Tyrosine Kinase Inhibitors and Increased Molecular Monitoring Frequency. *Journal of Managed Care & Specialty Pharmacy, 23*(2), 214-224.

Lehane, E., & McCarthy, G. (2007). Intentional and unintentional medication non-adherence: a comprehensive framework for clinical research and practice? A discussion paper. *International journal of nursing studies, 44*(8), 1468-1477.

Lowry, K. P., Dudley, T. K., Oddone, E. Z., & Bosworth, H. B. (2005). Intentional and unintentional nonadherence to antihypertensive medication. *Annals of Pharmacotherapy, 39*(7-8), 1198-1203.

Main, M., Kaplan, N., & Cassidy, J. (1985). Security in infancy, childhood, and adulthood: A move to the level of representation. *Monographs of the society for research in child development*, 66-104.

Martin, C. M. (2007). Chronic disease and illness care Adding principles of family medicine to address ongoing health system redesign. *Canadian Family Physician, 53*(12), 2086-2091.

Maslow, A. H. (1943). *A theory of human motivation. Psychological review*, 50(4), 370.

Maunder, R. G., & Hunter, J. J. (2009). Assessing patterns of adult attachment in medical patients. *General hospital psychiatry, 31*(2), 123-130.

Maunder, R., & Hunter, J. (2015). Love, fear, and health: how our attachments to others shape health and health care. *University of Toronto Press*.

Meredith, P. J., Strong, J., & Feeney, J. A. (2005). Evidence of a relationship between adult attachment variables and appraisals of chronic pain. *Pain Research and Management, 10*(4), 191-200.

Mikulincer, M., & Florian, V. The relationship between adult attachment styles and emotional and cognitive reactions to stressful events. In:

Simpson, J.A, Rholes, W.S., eds. *Attachment Theory and Close Relationships* (1998). New York: Guilford Press. 143-65.

Mikulincer, M., & Shaver, P. R. (2007). *Attachment in adulthood: Structure, dynamics, and change*. Guilford Press.

Mikulincer, M., Shaver, P. R., & Pereg, D. (2003). Attachment theory and affect regulation: The dynamics, development, and cognitive consequences of attachment-related strategies. *Motivation and Emotion, 27*, 77–102.

Murray, C. J., Vos, T., Lozano, R., Naghavi, M., Flaxman, A. D., Michaud, C., ... & Aboyans, V. (2013). Disability-adjusted life years (DALYs) for 291 diseases and injuries in 21 regions, 1990–2010: a systematic analysis for the Global Burden of Disease Study 2010. *The lancet, 380*(9859), 2197-2223.

Niederhauser, R. K. (2001). Adult attachment styles in primary care clinics for the medically underserved. *Dissertation Abstracts International: Section B: The Sciences and Engineering, 61*, 6716.

Obegi, J. H., & Berant, E. (Eds.). (2010). *Attachment theory and research in clinical work with adults*. Guilford press.

Özpolat, A. G. Y., Ayaz, T., Konağ, Ö., & Özkan, A. (2014). Attachment style and perceived social support as predictors of biopsychosocial adjustment to cancer. *Turkish journal of medical sciences, 44*(1), 24-30.

Paone, E., Pierro, L., Damico, A., Aceto, P., Campanile, F. C., Silecchia, G., & Lai, C. (2017). Alexithymia and weight loss in obese patients underwent laparoscopic sleeve gastrectomy. *Eating and Weight Disorders-Studies on Anorexia, Bulimia and Obesity*, 1-6.

Pasma, A., Schenk, C., Timman, R., van't Spijker, A., Appels, C., van der Laan, W. H., ... & Busschbach, J. J. (2017). Does non-adherence to DMARDs influence hospital-related healthcare costs for early arthritis in the first year of treatment? *PloS one, 12*(2), e0171070.

Peleg, S., Vilchinsky, N., Fisher, W., Khaskia, A., & Mosseri, M. (2016). Personality makes a difference: attachment orientation moderates theory of planned behaviour prediction of medication adherence. *European Health Psychologist, 18*(S), 660.

Raebel, M. A., Schmittdiel, J., Karter, A. J., Konieczny, J. L., & Steiner, J. F. (2013). Standardizing terminology and definitions of medication adherence and persistence in research employing electronic databases. *Medical care, 51*(8 0 3), S11.

Ravitz, P., Maunder, R., Hunter, J., Sthankiya, B., & Lancee, W. (2010). Adult attachment measures: A 25-year review. *Journal of psychosomatic research, 69*(4), 419-432.

Roebuck, M. C., Liberman, J. N., Gemmill-Toyama, M., & Brennan, T. A. (2011). Medication adherence leads to lower health care use and costs despite increased drug spending. *Health affairs, 30*(1), 91-99.

Rubenstein, C., & Shaver, P. R. (1982). *In search of intimacy: surprising conclusions from a nationwide survey on loneliness & what to do about it.* Delacorte Press.

Salander, P. (2002). Bad news from the patient's perspective: an analysis of the written narratives of newly diagnosed cancer patients. *Social science & medicine, 55*(5), 721-732.

Salari, A., Hasandokht, T., Mahdavi-Roshan, M., Kheirkhah, J., Gholipour, M., & Tootkaoni, M. P. (2016). Risk factor control, adherence to medication and follow up visit, five years after coronary artery bypass graft surgery. *Journal of cardiovascular and thoracic research, 8*(4), 152.

Salmon, P., & Young, B. (2009). Dependence and caring in clinical communication: the relevance of attachment and other theories. *Patient education and counseling, 74*(3), 331-338.

Say, R., Murtagh, M., & Thomson, R. (2006). Patients' preference for involvement in medical decision making: a narrative review. *Patient education and counseling, 60*(2), 102-114.

Shaver, P., & Rubenstein, C. (1980). Childhood attachment experience and adult loneliness. *Review of personality and social psychology, 1*, 42-73.

Simpson, J.A., Rholes, W. S. (1994). Stress and secure base relationships in adulthood. *Adv Person Rel, 5*, 181-204.

Sirois, F. M., & Gick, M. L. (2016). An appraisal-based coping model of attachment and adjustment to arthritis. *Journal of health psychology, 21*(5), 821-831.

Sperling, M. B., & Berman, W. H. (Eds.). (1994). *Attachment in adults: Clinical and developmental perspectives.* Guilford Press.

Tan, A., Zimmermann, C., & Rodin, G. (2005). Interpersonal processes in palliative care: an attachment perspective on the patient-clinician relationship. *Palliative Medicine, 19*(2), 143-150.

Thompson, D., & Ciechanowski, P. S. (2003). Attaching a new understanding to the patient-physician relationship in family practice. *The Journal of the American Board of Family Practice, 16*(3), 219-226.

Tonioni, F., D'Alessandris, L., Lai, C., Martinelli, D., Corvino, S., Vasale, M., ... & Bria, P. (2012). Internet addiction: hours spent online, behaviors and psychological symptoms. *General Hospital Psychiatry, 34*(1), 80-87.

Tryphonopoulos, P. D., Letourneau, N., & Ditommaso, E. (2014). Attachment and Caregiver–Infant Interaction: A Review of Observational-Assessment Tools. *Infant Mental Health Journal, 35*(6), 642-656.

van Dijk, L., Heerdink, E. R., Somai, D., van Dulmen, S., Sluijs, E. M., de Ridder, D. T., ... & Bensing, J. M. (2007). Patient risk profiles and practice variation in nonadherence to antidepressants, antihypertensives and oral hypoglycemics. *BMC health services research, 7*(1), 51.

van Dulmen, S., & van Bijnen, E. (2011). What makes them (not) talk about proper medication use with their patients? An analysis of the determinants of GP communication using reflective practice. *International Journal of Person Centered Medicine, 1*(1), 27-34.

van IJzendoorn, M. H. (1995). Adult attachment representations, parental responsiveness, and infant attachment: A meta-analysis on the predictive validity of the Adult Attachment Interview. *Psychological bulletin, 117*(3), 387.

Vilchinsky, N., Dekel, R., Revenson, T.A., Liberman, G., & Mosseri, M. (2015). Cardiac caregivers' burden and depressive symptoms: The moderational role of attachment orientations. *Health Psychology, 34*, 262–269.

Vrtička, P., Andersson, F., Grandjean, D., Sander, D., & Vuilleumier, P. (2008). Individual attachment style modulates human amygdala and striatum activation during social appraisal. *PLoS One, 3*(8), e2868.

Weiss, R. S. (1982). Attachment in adult life. In Parkes, CM, & Stevenson-Hinde, J. (Eds.), *The place of attachment in human behavior.*

Weiss, R. S. (1991). The attachment bond in childhood and adulthood. *Attachment across the life cycle, 8,* 66-76.

West, M. L. (1994). *Patterns of relating: An adult attachment perspective.* Guilford Press.

World Health Organization. (2017). *Chronic diseases and health promotion.* Retrieved from: http://www.who.int/chp/en/.

World Health Organization. (2017). *Noncommunicable diseases.* Retrieved from: http://www.who.int/mediacentre/factsheets/ fs355/en/.

Wright, E. B., Holcombe, C., & Salmon, P. (2004). Doctors' communication of trust, care, and respect in breast cancer: qualitative study. *Bmj, 328*(7444), 864.

Zhan, Y., Guo, Y., & Lu, Q. (2016). Aberrant Epigenetic Regulation in the Pathogenesis of Systemic Lupus Erythematosus and Its Implication in Precision Medicine. *Cytogenetic and genome research, 149*(3), 141-155.

In: Advances in Health and Disease
Editor: Lowell T. Duncan

ISBN: 978-1-53613-020-1
© 2018 Nova Science Publishers, Inc.

Chapter 5

HIP DISLOCATION: TYPES, CAUSES AND TREATMENTS

Alessandro Aprato, MD*, Michele Nardi, MD, Marco Favuto, MD, Gabriele Cominetti, MD, Kristijan Zoccola MD and Alessandro Massè MD
Orthopaedic Departement, University of Turin, Turin, Italy

ABSTRACT

Hip dislocation or subluxation may appear in a wide range of settings: it may result from traumatic injury, atraumatic capsular laxity, structural bony abnormality (such as acetabular dysplasia) and iatrogenic injury.

Traumatic hip dislocations, most often caused by motor vehicle accidents or similar high-energy impacts, traverse a large subset of distinct injury patterns. Non-surgical treatment is often recommended if no other associated injuries occurred while surgical treatment may be required in selected cases and may be performed arthroscopically or trough open surgery.

Dislocation may also occur after a minor trauma; in those cases often a predisposing anatomy is the leading cause of the instability. Treatment is controversial in those scenarios but surgeon should evaluate the femoral

---

[*] Corresponding Author E-mail: ale_aprato@hotmail.com.

and acetabular anatomy and, if indicated, offer its possible correction such as periacetabular osteotomy and/or femoral osteotomy.

Atraumatic subluxation of the hip is often present in patients with developmental dysplasia of the hip. The latter involves a spectrum of hip disorders that affect hip anatomy and development and can range from mild anatomical deformity with a reduced but subluxable hip to a frankly dislocated hip.

Eventually hip dislocation or subluxation may occur after surgical procedure and they have been reported after either hip arthroscopy either open procedures. In those cases, treatment is controversial and often ends in a total hip replacement.

In this chapter, the patterns of dislocation and subluxation are reviewed and their associated issue are described in order to allow surgeons to provide optimal care for these patients.

Keywords: hip disloaction, acetabulum, arthroscopy, Thompson-Epstein

INTRODUCTION

The hip is a ball-and-socket joint in which the head is incompletely covered. Due to the depth of the acetabulum (enhanced by the labrum), its thick capsule, and strong muscular support, the hip joint is less likely to dislocate when is compared to other joints in the body. The capsule is reinforced by strong capsular ligaments. The iliofemoral ligament, or Y ligament of Bigelow, is located anteriorly. The ischiofemoral ligament is located posteriorly. Eventually, the short external rotators adhere to the capsule posteriorly, providing additional stability.

In addition to the static stabilizers of the hip (capsular ligaments, bony anatomy), three muscles contribute to stability acting as dynamic stabilizers: the gluteus minimus, the reflected head of rectus femoris and iliocapsularis. These muscles have reproducible footprints on the capsule [1].

Hip dislocation and subluxation may result from several causes. High energy trauma may lead to traumatic hip dislocation. Sometimes fracture of hip joint may be associated. Low energy trauma may also cause dislocation of the hip but they are generally associated to predisposing anatomic conditions.

On the other hand atraumatic instability does not have a clear inciting event and it can originate from overuse, generalized dysplasia of the hip, hypermobility with capsular laxity or it can be impingement induced [2]. Eventually, hip dislocation or subluxation may occur as a complication after either open either arthroscopic surgical procedures.

High Energy Traumatic Dislocation

Hip dislocations have been reported in medical literature since the early nineteenth century. Several studies showed that most hip dislocation, 46% to 84% occur secondary to traffic accidents [3]. Associated acetabular fractures were seen in 70% of patients with traumatic hip dislocations, other lower extremity fractures in 23%, upper extremity fractures in 21%, closed head injuries in 24%, thoracic injuries in 21%, and abdominal injuries in 15% [3]. Another commonly associated injury is peripheral nerve injury. Cornwall and Radomisli reported a 10% incidence of nerve injury after traumatic hip dislocation [4].

With hip dislocations, the capsule is usually disrupted. Labral tears and muscular injury can occur as well. With an anterior hip dislocation, the iliopsoas tendon is a fulcrum for the hip, and the capsule is disrupted anteriorly and inferiorly. Posterior hip dislocations result in a tear through the posterior capsule. The Y ligament of Bigelow usually remains intact, and the capsule is stripped from its acetabular posterior attachment.

The mechanism of hip dislocation has been shown in multiple case studies to be axial loading, usually due to the impact with a dashboard in a motor vehicle crash [5]. Monma and Sugita proposed an alternative hypothesis to the dashboard mechanism of posterior dislocations [6]. They hypothesised the mechanism involved the vector force causing the dislocation is the pressure on the brake pedal with the right hip in a flexed, adducted, and internally rotated position.

Dislocation direction depends on hip position during trauma and the direction of the force vector applied, as well as the anatomy of the femur. Posterior dislocation (Figure 1) occurs after if sufficient force is applied on the long axis of the femoral shaft while the hip is flexed and adducted. In contrast, anterior dislocation occurs when the hip is abducted and externally rotated. Asymmetric dislocations are thought to be due to the different positions of the lower extremity during impact. Review of the literature reveals very few case reports of simultaneous asymmetric hips dislocations and most of these cases are result of "wind swept" position of the legs at the impact [7].

The classification system of Thompson-Epstein is the most commonly used. It has also a prognostic significance, as fractures associated with acetabular or femoral head fractures have worse prognoses than the others ones [8].

Posterior dislocation is more common than anterior one, the latter has an incidence between 9-24% [9].

Patients presenting with hip dislocation are unable to move the lower extremity and are in severe discomfort. The classic appearance of posterior hip dislocation is a patient with the hip in flexion, internal rotation, and adduction. Patients with an anterior dislocation hold the hip in marked external rotation, with mild flexion and abduction. Patients may have a palpable femoral head in the buttock region from a posterior dislocation or a femoral head prominence in the femoral triangle area with an anterior dislocation. A simple anteroposterior (AP) x-rays view of the pelvis is usually all that is needed to diagnose hip dislocations [10].

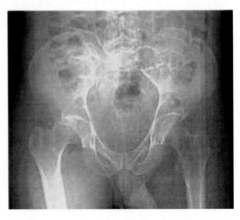

Figure 1. AP view of a posterior dislocation of the right hip.

Traumatic hip dislocations have significant long-term complications such as avascular necrosis (AVN) of the femoral head, early degenerative osteoarthritis, nerve impairment and heterotopic ossification. Associate injuries, time to reduction, direction of the dislocation, and general condition of the patient are the most reliable prognostic factors. In general, anterior dislocations without femoral head injury have a better long-term prognosis than posterior dislocations.

AVN is one of the most feared complications following hip dislocation. Previous studies have documented an osteonecrosis rate of 4.8% in patients who were reduced in less than 6 hours, whereas a 52.9% rate was seen in hips reduced after 6 hours from injury [11]. Although most of the authors agree that the risk of AVN increases when the hip remains dislocated for a longer period of time, some papers hypothesised that the incidence of AVN is not dependent on time until reduction, but rather the result of direct impact of the initial injury [12]. Although AVN is generally thought to occur within 2 years after hip dislocation, a recent report showed an AVN of the femoral head eight years after a posterior hip dislocation [11].

Post-traumatic arthritis is the most common complication in patients who have sustained a traumatic hip dislocation and probably results from articular cartilage injury during the initial dislocation (Figure 2). It occurred in up to 24% for simple dislocation and 88% for those associated with acetabular fracture [13].

Finally, recurrent dislocation following the index event is rare and is reported to occur only 1% of the time [14].

Low Energy Traumatic Dislocations

The normal hip is an inherently stable joint, and significant force is required to dislocate it. In rare cases hip dislocation may occur after a minor trauma. Hip dislocation after low energy trauma is more common in children. The flexible nature of soft tissues and bony structures and smaller sized hip joint (especially in children below age of five years) have been indicated as causes of dislocation without fracture. In healthy adult patients, anterior or posterior hip dislocation after low energy trauma have been descried in the literature as sporadic case. The etiology of this event is likely multifactorial and may be often associated with anatomic predisposition resulting from abnormal osseous morphology, generalized hyperlaxity, connective tissue disorders (such as Ehlers-Danlos syndrome, Marfan Syndrome, Down syndrome, Osteogenesis imperfecta) or repetitive microtrauma.

Recently there has been a resurgence of interest in proximal femoral anatomy because it has been theorized that subtle abnormalities in the bone anatomy can lead to damage of the soft tissue stabilizer of the hip, resulting in dislocation after minor trauma. Upadhayay et al. [16] attributed retroverted femoral neck to a predisposition to posterior dislocation of the hip joint. This deformity may cause repetitive micro trauma to the posterior soft tissue structures. Also significant coxa valga, long femoral neck and relatively anteverted bilateral femur can influence the stability of the hip [17]. Eventually an excessive retroversion of the acetabulum or insufficiency of the posterior wall may also lead to a posterior dislocation after minor trauma (Figure 3).

Stein et al. [18] and Epstein et al. [19] reported two cases of anterior hip dislocations after minor trauma in a dancer. The cause of these patient's dislocations were likely multifactorial. The osseous impingement at extreme ranges of motion may create levering of the femoral head, chondral shear injury ("contrecoup" injury), and end up in a subluxation or dislocation [20]. In a Philippon MJ et al. study, nine out of 14 patients with hip dislocations, were found to have underlying FAI [21]. Steppacher et al. in a comparative study, demonstrated a higher prevalence of radiographic markers associated with FAI in patients who sustained posterior hip dislocations compared with a group without instability [22]. These findings suggest that FAI may introduce an anatomic predisposition to posterior translation and subluxation, rendering these patients more prone to dislocation.

Low energy hip instability in the setting of normal osseous restraints has been considered rare. However, recent evidence suggests that attenuation of the hip's soft-tissue stabilizer may lead to development of microinstability.

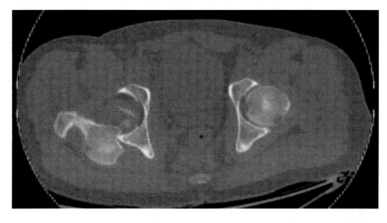

Figure 2. CT scan slice showing a cartilage lesion (Hill-sachs like) of the femoral head.

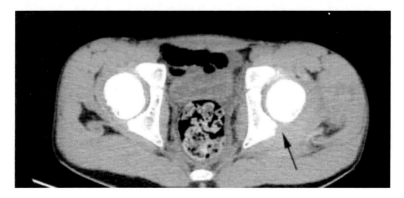

Figure 3. Ct scan slice of a 16 y.o. boy after reduction of a posterior low energy dislocation showing an insufficient posterior wall (arrow).

Overuse/microtraumatic injuries are common in athletes who participate to football, rugby, bicycling, skiing, dancing and hockey because it involved repetitive hip rotation with axial loading (e.g., Golf, figure skating, football, tennis, ballet, martial arts). The labrum or iliofemoral ligament may be damaged from these repetitive forces, increasing the translation or the femoral head relative to the acetabulum, stressing these structures (labrum and capsular ligament) even further. These abnormal forces cause increased tension in the joint capsule that can lead to painful labral injury, capsular redundancy and subsequent instability.

Atraumatic Hip Dislocation or Subluxation

In contrast to traumatic hip instability, which often involves an identifiable event or activity, atraumatic instability and subluxation do not have a clear inciting event and are associated with long standing anatomic abnormalities and general diseases.

Atraumatic instability can be divided into those of dysplastic and idiopathic origin. Dysplastic hip is any hip that had an abnormal development of the acetabular or/and the femoral components. Structural deformity of the dysplastic hip is complex and variable. It may also be caused by others diseases that affect the normal hip growth (Down syndrome, infantile cerebral palsy, Neurofibromatosis type 1, Ehelers - Danlos syndrome, Marfan sindorme, Stickler syndorme, Osteogenesis imperfecta type 1, Saul-Wilson Syndrome, myelomenigocele, Shprintzen sindorme [23]). The result is a wide spectrum of clinical conditions which may range from asymptomatic anatomical hip deformity to hip dislocation. DDH prevalence varies from 1.6 to 28.5 cases per 1000 children depending on the definition and the population being studied [24]. However, uncorrected DDH, especially when associated with hip dislocation, is associated with significant long term morbidity including gait abnormalities, chronic pain and premature degenerative arthritis requiring joint replacement in young age.

Acetabular deformity in dysplasia includes a shallow and abnormal inclined articular surface that provides decreased coverage of the femoral head (Figure 4). The acetabulum is often located in a slightly lateralized position. The femoral deformity may include coxa valga or increased femoral antiversion, both of which are variable. These combined deformities result in structural instability with overload of acetabular rim leading to labral and chondral injury and ultimately osteoarthritis [25].

Generally in DDH, the acetabulum presents an excessive antiversion from the sagittal plane [26] although Ganz [27] found that 7.2% of dysplasic hip has retroverted acetabulum. Furthermore his group have classified dysplastic acetabuli into two radiological types [28]: in the type 1 hip joints are radiologically incongruent while in type 2 are not congruent. In type 1, the acetabulum is more vertical than normal, swallow and has a diameter greater than that of the femoral head. In type 2, the acetabulum has a radius of curvature similar to that of the femoral head but it supplied less than normal cover for the femur.

In patients without the classic pattern of hip dysplasia, abnormal morphology of the acetabulum and the femoral head and neck may render the hip unstable and subluxable [29]. For example, patients with Legg Calvè Perthes disease may develop significant impingement that leads to secondary acetabular dysplasia and subsequent instability.

Hip instability and subluxation is common in children with cerebral palsy. It has been reported to occur in up to 83% of cases of spastic quadriplegia [30]. The incidence of spastic hip subluxation is associated with severity of neurological disorders, ambulatory function, and progresses with age and degrees of contracture. In addition to muscle imbalance and contracture, acetabular deficiency, excessive anteversion of the femur and coxa valga due to lack of physiological walking stress are also responsible for hip subluxation and dysplasia.

The direction of spastic hip subluxation is generally agreed to be lateral or posterolateral after adduction and flexion contracture of the hip [31].

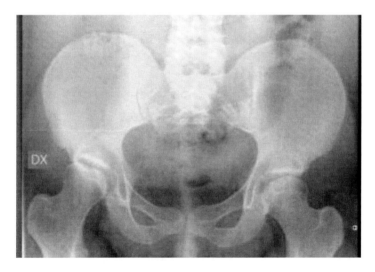

Figure 4. Ap pelvic view showing a severe dysplasia of the right hip and a mild dysplasia of the left hip.

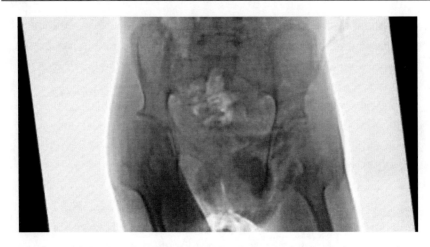

Figure 5. Ap pelvic view showing a severe dysplasia of the right hip in a 17 y.o boy with neurofibromatosis.

Hip instability and subluxation in children with Down syndrome have been described and prevalence has been reported at around 3% [32]. Instability may be due to joint laxity and acetabular retroversion but also muscles imbalance may have a role [33]. Soft-tissue disorders (such as generalized laxity) may also be responsible for hip instability. Ehlers - Danlos Syndrome is the most common connective tissue disorder causing generalized joint hypermobility. The latter predispose to instability and hip subluxation.

Neurofibromatosis type 1 (NF-1) also has been associated with hip deformity (Figure 5). The most common abnormalities include intraosseous cystic lesion, intra-articular neurofibromas, periostal bone proliferation, acetabular protusio coxa valga and increased femoral offset [34].

Atraumatic hip subluxation is a well-described entity in patients with joint hypermobility. Joint hypermobility is defined as supra physiologic range of motion in one or several joints [35]. In its simplest form, joint hypermobility is asymptomatic, and should be distinguished from Joint Hypermobility Syndrome (JHS) and other heritable disorders of connective tissue. JHS is a complex spectrum of signs and symptoms associated with the objective finding of joint hyperlaxity in absence of heritable disorders of connective tissue [36].

Iatrogenic Hip Instability

Hip instability may occur after surgical procedure and has been reported either after arthroscopic procedures either with open surgery [37].

Hip arthroscopy has experienced a considerable increase in popularity, largely resulting from improvements in techniques and technology. Rare but serious postoperative complications are instability and dislocation [38]. Arthroscopic postoperative instability is multifactorial, with both osseous and soft tissue contributions. Pre (minimal dysplasia, ligamentous laxity) and intraoperative factors (i.e., labral debridement, iliopsoas tenotomy, over-resection of acetabular rim, unrepaired capsulotomy, ligamentum teres debridement) may play a role in postoperative instability [37].

Capsular management during hip arthroscopy has been a significant subject of recent debate. Although some degree of capsular incision is necessary for visualization during arthroscopy, the capsule seems to play an important static role in joint stability and an excessive capsulotomy may lead to microinstability [39].

Preoperative acetabular undercoverage or iatrogenic over-resection of the acetabular rim (iatrogenic dysplasia) can create an environment susceptible to instability. Matsuda described a 39-year-old woman who underwent cam osteoplasty and excessive acetabular rim trimming (4 to 7 mm) and sustained a hip dislocation in the recovery room [40]. Souza et al. reported an anterior hip dislocation on the first port operative day following arthroscopic pincer decompression which the attributed to an excessive anterior rim resection [41]. Similarly, Benali et al. [42] reported excessive rim resection as the primary reason for postoperative hip dislocation.

Iliopsoas tendon is another important factor to the hip stability. Arthroscopic iliopsoas tendon release has been reported to be successful in athletes with painful hip snapping caused by the psoas tendon. However iliopsoas tenotomy may induce anterior microinstability, especially in presence of increased femoral anteversion [43].

Iatrogenic instability following a hip-preservation surgery is not exclusive to arthroscopic procedures (Figure 6-7). Instability following surgical hip dislocation or open procedures has also been described. Nepple et al. described a patient who presented with iatrogenic hip subluxation after undergoing a surgical hip dislocation with acetabuloplasy, labral refixation, and femoral osteochondroplasty for pincer impingement [44]. Due to ongoing symptoms and subluxation, the patient was successfully treated with periacetabular osteotomy.

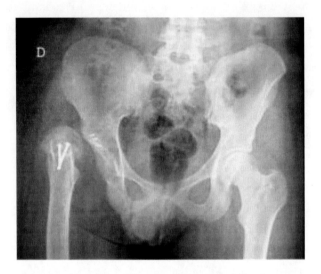

Figure 6. Ap pelvic view showing an anterior dislocation following an excessive anterior acetabular trimming via surgical safe dislocation.

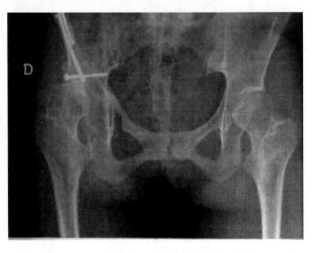

Figure 7. Ap pelvic view showing a femoral head subluxation following a poor coverage after periacetabular osteotomy.

Subluxation as a consequence of subcapital re-alignment for patients with slipped capital femoral epiphysis (SCFE) has also been reported [45]. We described three main groups of causes of instability in these patients. The first group includes causes directly related to SCFE: damage to the acetabular labrum, severe abrasion of acetabular cartilage and acetabular adaptation (flattening of acetabular roof). The second group includes causes not related to the SCFE as acetabular orientation and poor quality of the soft tissues. The third group includes causes directly related to surgical steps: neck shortening, insufficient trochanteric advancement and capsulotomy [46] in presence of other risk factors.

In summary, loss of congruity, instability and dislocation of the hip are potential complications of both open and arthroscopic surgical procedures. There are several reasons why this might occur. Some are related to the primary deformity but others are a consequence of the surgical intervention. Byrd et al. [47] described iatrogenic instability of the hip likely a perfect storm with enough factors coming together just wrong to create the problem. Intraoperative tests of stability should be part of the procedures because the best time for any additional measures to stabilise the hip is at the time of initial surgery.

EVALUATION

In acute cases of dislocation, anteroposterior and lateral Xray view is sufficient for the diagnosis. Post-reduction plain films should be performed to confirm a satisfactory reduction.

Following reduction maneuvers, or in the case of spontaneous reduction or subluxation, complementary plain radiographs should be acquired: true antero-posterior pelvis, lateral view of the proximal femur (Dunn or Frog Lateral) and false-profile view, These images, along with Judet oblique views of the pelvis, should be adequate to visualize any fractures, avulsions, loose bodies, nonconcentric reduction, recurrent subluxation or dislocation, or degenerative joint disease. In addition, acetabular coverage may be measured with central and lateral center edge angle respectively on anteroposterior and false-profile views. Several reports [19, 48] described those angles as the most useful indicator of instability.

Other helpful evaluation for dysplasia are the acetabular index [49], femoral head extrusion index, sharp angle [50] and the acetabular version. Cam impingement should also be documented, as it may be also associated with acetabular dysplasia.

Computed tomography (CT) scan is commonly performed in traumatic dislocation. The utility of the CT scan is to identify any posterior wall acetabular fractures, anterior or posterior or acetabular lip fractures, intra-articular loose bodies, or a nonconcentric reduction. Also, CT remains the gold standard for characterizing bony deformity.

In atraumatic cases, magnetic resonance imaging (MRI) was an important part of the evaluation of the hip. Although in the last decade [51] magnetic resonance imaging arthrography (MRA) has been indicated as the gold standard for assessment of labral, capsular and cartilage damage and deficiency.

In cases where diagnosis of instability is still in question, fluoroscopic examination under anesthesia may provide addition information [13].

TREATMENT

Trauma Cases

The treatment of an acute hip dislocation, regardless of causation of its, is early reduction. The urgency for reduction relates to the compromised blood flow to the femoral head and the risk of subsequent AVN, which varies in the literature from 11%-37% [52]. Reduction within 6 hours has been advocated to reduce the risk of developing AVN.

Once the diagnosis is made, urgent reduction is usually performed under general anesthesia.

Several techniques have been described for closed reduction [53]. Regardless of dislocation direction, the reduction may be attempted using in-line traction with the patient lying supine, followed by applying a force opposing the vector of the initial injury. Allis method, Stimson Gravity technique and Bigelow and Reverse Bigelow are the most common used.

Following closed reduction, post-reduction radiographs should be obtained to confirm adequate reduction followed by evaluation of post procedure neurovascular status. The hip should be examined for stability, while the patient is still sedated or under anesthesia.

If a displaced acetabular fracture is present or a posterior wall fragment greater than 33% is identified, stability examination may not be performed, as operative fixation is indicated.

On the other hand, open management is required for include irreducible dislocations and nonconcentric reductions with intra-articular fragments of bone or cartilage [54]. Roughly 2% to 15% of hip dislocations are irreducible [54].

Open reduction should be approached from the direction that the hip dislocated. Posterior dislocations are addressed via a Kocher-Langenbach approach. Anterior dislocations are addressed via an anterior (Smith-Petersen) or an anterolateral (Watson-Jones) approach. The operative approach is based on the associatedlesions and surgeon preference.

Excision of intra-articular of loose fragments, especially if the reduction is not concentric, is another indication for surgery (Figure 8) [55]. Fragments that require excision are interposed between the articular surfaces of the head and the acetabulum. Small fragments that are seen in the fovea and do not impinge on the head need not be removed. This finding is common and usually represents a small piece of bone avulsed from the femoral head by the ligamentum teres.

Hip arthroscopy has recently increased as a treatment modality for various conditions, including presence of loose bodies after hip dislocation. Small intra-articular fragments that do not require fixation may be removed arthroscopically and labral pathology addressed. The advantage of avoiding a large open incision and arthrotomy is apparent; however, the timing of arthroscopy is debated [56, 57].

In a series of 36 patients undergoing arthroscopy, 33 (92%) were found to have loose bodies. Interestingly, 7 of 8 (78%) patients who had a concentric reduction and no evidence of radiographic loose bodies were found to have intra-articular loose bodies at the time of arthroscopy [57].

Post reduction management is controversial. Some investigators recommend a temporary period of traction until the patient's initial pain has subsided, but this has not been proven beneficial. Most of surgeons recommend a period of touch weight bearing (TTWB) varying from 2-6 weeks although there is no agreement on this topic [58]. Traditionally, hip flexion to 90° and internal rotation to 10° is limited for 4 to 6 weeks to allow for capsular and soft-tissue healing.

At 6 weeks an MRI may be indicated to exclude an AVN [59].

At arrival, treatment of low energy hip dislocation is similar to the high energy cases. After reduction, treatment aim to bone deformity correction and/or soft tissue repair: derotational femoral osteotomy and/or acetabular osteotomy, open anterior or posterior capsulorhaphy should be considered on the base of the supposed causes of instability.

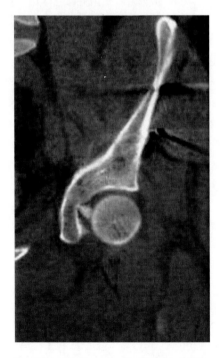

Figure 8. Ct scan slice showing an intra-articular fragment after reduction of a posterior dislocation.

Atraumatic Cases

Dysplastic patients benefit from corrective osteotomies of the acetabulum and/or proximal femur in the earliest stages [60]. The acetabular deformity remains the most commonly treated component of hip dysplasia. The most appropriate type of pelvic osteotomy is chosen evaluating patient's age and deformity type.

In the past, procedures such as the Chiari osteotomy or shelf augmentation of the acetabulum would be used to treat adolescent and adult hip dysplasia. In the last decade, Bernese periacetabular osteotomy (PAO) [60] became the preferred technique in North America and Europe for acetabular reorientation [61]. Zaltz et al. [62] reported the safety of PAO among experienced surgeons with major complication rate 5.9%.

PAO should aim to provide normalization of coverage, but also normalization of the version. In particular understanding acetabular version is essential to perform the correction. In most cases of acetabular dysplasia, the deficit is anterolateral and the surgeon therefore rotates the acetabular fragment foreword and laterally [27].

Indications for PAO included a patient with a dysplastic hip with symptoms for more than five months, a lateral centre edge angle of Wiberg of <16° on AP radiographs, and an improvement of joint congruency on an AP radiograph in abduction [63]. Contraindications are: presence of hip dislocation, the presence of a secondary acetabulum, lost of articular congruence in the anteroposterior view with the leg abducted and advanced arthritis.

Acetabular deformity is the most treated portion of the deformity in this patient population but some patients with hip dysplasia have a femoral predominant deformity. A derotational femoral osteotomy may normalize underlying femoral deformity. Several technique for derotational osteotomy have been described with successful results [61].

Total hip arthroplasty (THA) is the best option of care in advanced arthritis and literature offers a clear evidence for this statement. That said, young age and distorted anatomy are bad prognostic factors for long term survival of THA [62].

Iatrogenic hip instability treatment is not clear at present. Instability due to capsulotomy may be treated with arthroscopic reconstruction of the IFL [67] or reconstruction of the anterior capsule [68] with iliotibial band autograft although these treatments remain controversial. When ligamentum teres was thought to be the main cause of instability, reconstruction of the ligament has been performed although up to date survival of the reconstructed ligament has not been documented [69]. If iatrogenic hip instability is related to bone deformity, acetabular and/or femoral correction osteotomies may be considered. In case of either severe hip pain or persistent hip instability after surgical procedures, aimed at correcting the iatrogenic instability itself, and also in case of severe osteoarthritis patients should undergo THA.

REFERENCES

[1] Walters BL, Cooper JH, Rodriguez JA. New findings in hip capsular anatomy: Dimensions of capsular thickness and pericapsular contributions. *Arthroscopy*. 2014; 30 (10): 1235-1245.

[2] Domb BG, Philippon MJ, Giordano BD. Arthroscopic capsulotomy, capsular repair, and capsular plication of the hip: Relation to atraumatic instability. *Arthroscopy*. 2013; 29: 162-173.

[3] Hak DJ, Goulet JA. Severity of injuries associated with traumatic hip dislocation as a result of motor veichle collisions. *J. Trauma*. 1999; 47 (1): 60-3.

[4] Cornwall R, Radomisli TE. Nerve injury in traumatic dislocation of the hip. *Clin. Orthop. Rel. Res.* 2000; (377): 84-91.

[5] Kundu ZS, Mittal R, Sangwan SS, Sharma A. Simultaneous asymmetric bilateral hip dislocation with unilateral fracture of the femur-peculiar mode of trauma in a case. *Eur. J. Orthop. Surg. Traumatol*. 2003; 13: 255-7.

[6] Monma H, Sugita T. Is the mechanism of traumatic posterior dislocation of the hip a brake pedal injury rather than a dashboard injury? *Injury*. 2001; 32 (3): 221-2.

[7] Bilsel K, Alpan B, Ugutmen E et al. Bilateral simultaneous traumatic hip dislocation in opposite directions: a case report. *Acta Orthop. Belg.* 2009; 75(2):270-2.

[8] Bucholz RW, Wheeless G. Irreducible posterior fracture dislocations of the hip. The role of the iliofemoral ligament and the rectus femoris muscle. *Clin. Orthop. Relat. Res.* 1982; Jul(167): 118-22.

[9] Alonso JE, Volgas DA, Giordano V, Stannard JP. A review of the treatment of hip dislocations associated with acetabular fractures. *Clin. Orthop. Rel. Res.* 2000; (377): 32-43.

[10] Tornetta P, Hamid MR. Hip dislocation: current treatment regimens. *J. Am. Acad. Orthop. Surg.* 1997; 5: 27-36.

[11] Cash DJW, Nolan JF. Avascular necrosis of the femoral head 8 years after posterior hip dislocation. *Injury.* 2007; 38: 865-7.

[12] Browner BD, Jupiter J, Levine AM, Trafton PG, Krettek C, editors. *Skeletal trauma.* 4th ed. Philadelphia: WB Saunders; 2009.

[13] David M. Foulk, Brian H. Mullis. Hip dislocation: evaluation and management. *J. Am. Acad. Ortoph. Surg.* 2010; 18: 199-209.

[14] Rockwood Jr CA, Green DP, Bucholz R. *Fractures in adults.* 4th ed. Philadelphia: Lippincott-Raven; 1996.

[15] Bosch AM, Hammacher ER, Van der Werken C. Recurrent traumatic dislocation of the hip joint at the age of 13 and 17 years. A case reports. *Acta Orthop. Belg.* 2000; 66 (2): 187-199.

[16] Upadhayay SS, Moulton A, Burwell RG. Biological factors predisposing to posterior dislocation of the hip. *J. Bone Joint Surf. Br.* 1985; 67 (2): 548.

[17] Crawford Mj, Dy Cj, Alexander JW, Thompson M, Schroder SJ, Vega CE, Patel RV, Miller AR, McCarthy JC, Lowe WR, Noble PC. The biomechanics of the hip labrum and the stability of the hip. *Clin. Orthop. Relat. Res.* 2007; 465:16-22.

[18] Stein Da, Poltasch DB, Giudumal R, Rose DJ. Low-energy anterior hip dislocation in a dancer. *Am. J. rthop.* 2002; 31(10): 591-594.

[19] David M. Epstein, Donald J. Rose, Marc J. Philippon. Arthroscopic Management of Recurrent Low Energy Anterior Hip Dislocation in Dancer, a case report. *The American Journal of Sports Medicine*, Vol 38, No. 6.

[20] Beatrice Shu, Marc R. Safran. Hip instability; anatomic and clinical considerations of traumatic and atraumatic instarbility. *Clin. Sports Med.* 2011; 30: 349-367.

[21] Philippon MJ, Kuppersmith DA, Wolff AB, Briggs KK. Artroscopic findings following traumatic hip dislocation in 14 professional athletes. *Arthroscopy.* 2009; 25 (2): 169-174.

[22] Steppacher SD, Albers CE, Siebenrock KA, Tannas M, Ganz R. Femoroacetabular impingement predisposes to traumatic posterior hip dislocation. *Clin. Orthop. Relat. Res.* 2013; 471(6):1937-43.

[23] Jonathan C. Riboh, Jeffrey Grzybowski, Richard C. Mather III, Shane J. Nho. A traumatic Hip Instability in Patients with Joint Hypermobility. *Operative techniques in sport medicine.* 2015; 23 (3): 203-212.

[24] V Bialik, GM Bialik, S Blazer, P Sujov, F Wiener. Developmental dysplasia of the hip: a new approach to incidence. *Pediatrics.* 1999; 103 (1):93-9.

[25] Jeffrey J, Nepple MD, John Clohisy MD. The dysplastic and unstable hip: a responsible balance of arthroscopic and open approaches. *Sports Med. Arthrosc. Rev.* 2015; 23 (4): 180-6.

[26] Salter RB. Innominate osteotomy in the treatment of congenital dislocation of the hip. *J. Bone Joint Surg.* 1961; 43B: 518-539.

[27] Patrick L.S. Li, MD; and Reinhold Ganz, MD. Morphologic Features of Congenital Acetabular Dysplasia: One in Six is Retroverted. *Clinical Orthopeadics and related research.* 2003; 416: 245-253.

[28] K. Klaue, C. W. Durnin, R. Ganz. The acetabular rim syndrome a clinical presentation of dysplasia of the hip. *J. Bone Joint Surg.* 1991; 73-B: 423-9.

[29] Ganz R, Parvizi J, Beck M, Leunig M, Notzli H, Siebenrock KA. Femoro acerabular impingement: a cause of osteoarthritis of the hip. *Clin. Orthop. Relat. Res.* 2003; (417) 112-120.

[30] Abel MF, Wenger DR, Mubarak SJ et al. Quantitative analysis of hip dysplasia in cerebral palsy: a study of radiographs and 3-D reformatted images. *J. Pediatr. Orthop.* 1994; 14:283-289.

[31] Lonstein JE, Beck K. Hip dislocation and subluxation in cerebral palsy. *J. Pediatr. Orthop.* 1986; 6: 521-526.

[32] Bennet GC, Rang M, Roye DP et al. Dislocation of the hip in trisomy 21. *J. Bone Joint Surg. Br.* 1982; 64: 289-294.

[33] Eshuis R, Boonzaaijer M, van Weiringen H et al. Assessment of the relationship between joint laxity and migration of the hip in children with Down syndrome. *J. Child Orthop.* 2012; 6:373-377.

[34] Paul M. Dearden, Kathryn A. Lowery, Joanna Bates, Sandeep P. Datir. Hip dislocation following minor trauma in a patient with NF-1: a case report and review of the literature. *Hip Int.* 2015 25(2): 188-190.

[35] Hakim A, Grahame R: Joint hypermobility. *Best Pract. Res. Clin. Rheumatol.* 2003; 17(6): 989-1004.

[36] Bird HA. Joint hypermobility. *Musculoskeletal Care.* 2007; 5(1):4-19.

[37] Neil L. Duplantier, M.D., Patrick C. McCulloch, M.D., Shane J. Nho, M.D., Richard C. Mather III, M.D., Brian D. Lewis, M.D., and Joshua D. Harris, M.D. Hip Dislocation or Subluxation After Hip Arthroscopy: A Systematic Review. *Arthroscopy.* 2016 Jul; 32 (7): 1428-34.

[38] Clarke MT, Villar RN. Hip arthroscopy: complications in 1054 cases. *Clin. Orthop.* 2003; 406: 84-88.

[39] Harris J, Gerrie B, Lintner D, Varner K, McCulloch P. Microinstability of the hip and the splits X-ray. *Orthopedics.* 2016; 39:1-6.

[40] Matsuda DK. Acute iatrogenic dislocation following hip impingement arthroscopic surgery. *Arthroscopy.* 2009; 25:400-404.

[41] Souza BG, Dani WS, Honda EK, Ricioli W jr, Guimaraes RP, Ono Nk, Polesello GC. Do complication in hip arthroscopy change with experience? *Arthroscopy.* 2010 26 (8): 1053-7.

[42] Benali Y, Katthagen BD. Hip subluxation as a complication of arthroscopic debridement. *Arthroscopy.* 2009 Apr; 25(4):405-7.

[43] Nikolaos V. Bardakos. Hip impingement: beyond femoroacetabular. *J. Hip. Preserv. Surg.* 2015; 2(3): 206-223.

[44] Nepple JJ, Schoenecker P, Clohisy J. Iatrogenic hip subluxation after surgical dislocation successfully treated with periacetabular osteotomy: a case report. *JBJS Case Connect.* 2013 9; 3 (1).
[45] Ganz R, Aprato A, Mazziotta G, Pignatti G. Joint instability after anatomic reconstruction of severe, chronic SCFE. A Report of 3 Cases, with High Femoral Anteversion in 1 and Adaptive Acetabular Roof Deformation in 3. *JBJS Case Connect.* 2016; 6:50.
[46] Ganz R, Gill TJ, Gautier E et al. Safe surgical dislocation of the adult hip. *J. Bone Joint Surg.* 2001; 83: 1119-1124.
[47] J. W. Thomas Byrd, M.D. Iatrogenic Instability of the Hip: A Perfect Storm. *Arthroscopy: The Journal of Arthroscopic and Related Surgery.* 2016; 32 (6): 1205-1206.
[48] Maeyama A, Naito M, Moriyama S, Yoshimura I. Evaluation of dynamic instability of the dysplastic hip with use of triaxial accelerometry. *J. Bone Joint Surg.* 2008; 90 (1): 85-92.
[49] Lequesne M: Coxometrie: Mesure des angles fondamentaux de la hanche radiographique de l'adulte par un rapporteur combine [Coxometry: Measurement of the fundamental angles of the adult radiographic hip by a combined protractor]. *Rev. Rhum.* 1936; 30:479-485.
[50] Sharp IK. Acetabular dysplasia, the acetabular angle. *J. Bone Joint Surg.* 1961; 43-B: 268-72.
[51] Leunig M, Werlen S, Ungersbock A, Ito K, Ganz R: Evaluation of the acetabular labrum by MR arthrography. *J. Bone Joint Surg.* 79B:230-234, 1997.
[52] Sahin V, Karakaş ES, Aksu S, Atlihan D, Turk CY, Halici M. Traumatic dislocation and fracture-dislocation of the hip: a long-term follow-up study. Dislocation of the hip: A long-term follow-up study. *J. Trauma.* 2003 Mar; 54(3):520-9.
[53] Sharma S, Kumar V, Dhillon MS: A new technique for closed reduction of traumatic posterior dislocations of the hip: The 'PGI technique.' *Hip Int.* 2014. 24:394-398.
[54] Tornetta P, Mostafavi H. Hip Dislocation: Current Treatment Regimens. *J. Am. Acad. Orthop. Surg.* 1997; 5(1):27-36.

[55] Levine RG, Kauffman CP, Reilly MC, Behrens FF. 'Floating pelvis.' A combination of bilateral hip dislocation with a lumbar ligamentous disruption. *J. Bone Joint Surg. Br.* 1999; 81(2):309-11.

[56] Chernchujit B, Sanguanjit P, Arunakul M. Arthroscopic loose body removal after hip fracture dislocation: Experiences in 7 cases. *J. Med. Assoc. Thai.* 2009; 92: 161-164.

[57] Mullis BH, Dahners LE. Hip arthroscopy to remove loose bodies after traumatic dislocation. *J. Orthop. Trauma.* 2006; 20:22-26.

[58] Shu B, Safran MR. Hip instability: Anatomic and clinical considerations of traumatic and atraumatic instability. *Clin. Sports Med.* 2011; 30: 349-367.

[59] Shindle MK, Ranawat AS, Kelly BT: Diagnos is and management of traumatic and atraumatic hip instability in the athletic patient. *Clin. Sports Med.* 2006;25:309-326.

[60] Ganz R, Klaue K, Vinh TS, Mast JW: A new periacetabular osteotomy for the treatment of hip dysplasia: Technique and preliminary results. *Clin. Orthop.* 1988; 232: 26-36.

[61] Jeffrey J, Nepple MD, John Clohisy MD. The dysplastic and ustable hip: a responsible balance of arthroscopic and open approaches. *Sports Med. Arthrosc. Rev.* 2015; 23 (4): 180-6.

[62] Zaltz I. Baca G, Kim YJ et al. Complications associated with the periacetabular osteotomy: a prospective multicenter study. *J. Bone Joint Surf., Am. Case Reports.* 2014; 96:1967-1974.

[63] Naito M, Shiramizu K, Akiyoshi Y, Ezoe M, Nakamura Y. Curved periacetabular osteotomy for treatment of dysplastic hip. *Clin. Orthop.* 2005; 433: 129-35.

[64] Stefanie N. Hofstede, Maaike G. J. Gademan, Thea P. M. Vliet Vlieland, Rob G. H. H. Nelissen and Perla J. Marang-van de Mheen. Preoperative predictors for outcomes after total hip replacement in patients with osteoarthritis: a systematic review. *BMC Musculoskeletal Disorders.* 2012; 17: 212.

[65] Emilios E. Pakos Nikolaos K. Paschos, Theodoros A. Xenakis. Long Term Outcomes of Total Hip Arthroplasty in Young Patients under 30. *Arch. Bone Jt. Surg.* 2014 Sep; 2(3): 157-162.

[66] Omer Mei-Dan, M.D., Tigran Garabekyan, M.D., Mark McConkey, M.D., and Cecilia Pascual-Garrido, M.D. Arthroscopic Anterior Capsular Reconstruction of the Hip for Recurrent Instability. *Arthroscopy Techniques*. 2015; 4 (6): 711-715.

[67] Dierckman BD, Guanche CA. Anterior hip capsule ligamentous reconstruction for recurrent instability after hip arthroscopy. *Am. J. Orthop.* 2014; 43: 319-323.

[68] De SA D, Phillips M, Philippon MJ et al. Ligamentum teres injuries of the hip: a systematic review examining surgical indications, treatment options, and outcomes. *Arthroscopy*. 2014; 30: 1634-1641.

In: Advances in Health and Disease
Editor: Lowell T. Duncan

ISBN: 978-1-53613-020-1
© 2018 Nova Science Publishers, Inc.

Chapter 6

MULTICENTRIC CASTLEMAN DISEASE: ASSOCIATED AND DIFFERENTIAL DISORDERS

Yoshinori Tanino[*] and Hiroyuki Minemura
Department of Pulmonary Medicine, Fukushima Medical University
School of Medicine, Fukushima-City, Fukushima, Japan

ABSTRACT

Castleman's disease (CD) is a rare lymphoproliferative syndrome, and is derived into two groups: unicentric and multicentric. Unicentric Castleman's disease is presented as an isolated mass, such as mediastitial lymph node, and is curable with surgery in most cases. Multicentric Castleman's disease (MCD) is comprised of heterogeneous disorders with various etiologies and represents systemic inflammatory symptoms, such as fever and weight loss. Human herpes virus-8 (HHV-8) is thought to be a causable pathogen in all HIV-positive MCD patients, as well as some HIV-negative MCD patients, via hypercytokinemia. Definitive diagnosis

---

[*] Corresponding Author Tel: (+81)24-547-1360, Fax: (+81) 24-548-9366, E-mail: ytanino@fmu.ac.jp.

of MCD is difficult because a variety of disorders, such as malignancy, inflammatory and infectious diseases, represent MCD-like features. Recently, the term, idiopathic MCD (iMCD) has been proposed as HHV-8-negative MCD by the international, evidence-based consensus diagnostic criteria. Although the diagnostic criteria requires to exclude various disorders which show similar clinical characteristics as MCD to make a diagnosis of iMCD, it is difficult to differentiate these similar disorders such as malignant lymphoma, autoimmune diseases, POEMS syndrome, IgG4-related disease, autoimmune lymphoproliferative syndrome (ALPS) and virus infection from MCD. In addition, there has been an intense debate on the difference between the disorders and MCD. That is, it has not been clarified if MCD is exactly different from these disorders or is the associated clinical phenotype of them. We recently reported a case of MCD with ALPS, which is a rare nonmalignant lymphoproliferative disorder characterized by increase in CD3+TCR$\alpha\beta$+CD4-CD8- double-negative T (DNT) cells and peripheral lymphadenopathy. We herein discuss the association and difference between MCD and various disorders that represent MCD-like features.

Keywords: Castleman's disease, multicentric Castleman's disease, HHV-8, IL-6, Autoimmune lymphoproliferative syndrome

1. INTRODUCTION

1.1. Castleman's Disease (CD)

CD was first described in 1956 by Dr. Benjamin Castleman, who reported that the disease was characterized by unicentric lymphadenopathy with hyperplastic lymphoid tissue and hyalinized germinal centers [1]. Because the enlarged lymph node is localized, this CD type was referred to as unicentric CD (UCD). The histological findings of the involved lymph node in UCD are the hyaline-vascular lesions characterized by small hyaline-vascular follicles and interfollicular capillary proliferation (i.e., hyaline vascular type). The treatment of UCD, which is usually curable, consists of surgical resection and has a good prognosis in most patients [2].

In 1984, hypervascular follicular hyperplasia was described in a patient with AIDS [3]. Later, a number of reports described the presence of lymphadenopathy in more than one affected region, together with CD-like features, in HIV-positive patients [4]. In most of these patients, the histological findings of the affected lymph nodes are plasma cell lesions characterized by large follicles with intervening sheets of plasma cells (i.e., plasma cell type) or a mixed type of both hyaline-vascular and plasma-cell types [5]. These cases were referred to as multicentric CD (MCD), and CD was subsequently separated into two groups: UCD and MCD [6, 7].

Here, we review the recent understanding of CD. In addition, we describe a case of MCD with autoimmune lymphoproliferative syndrome (ALPS) and discuss the possible association of MCD with ALPS.

1.2. Multicentric Castleman's Disease (MCD)

Patients with MCD display systemic inflammatory symptoms, such as fever, weight loss, night sweats, edema, ascites, pleural effusions, and splenomegaly [7]. Histopathological findings of multifocal lymphadenopathy reveal characteristic features [5, 7]. Pathological findings of MCD are usually consistent with plasma cell or mixed types [6]. During the HIV pandemic, human herpes virus 8 (HHV-8) [or Kaposi's sarcoma (KS)-associated herpesvirus] was reported to be casually linked to the etiology of HIV-positive and -negative MCD [8–10]. HHV-8 replication causes viral-dependent hypercytokinemia and is considered to be responsible for the clinicopathological findings of MCD, regardless of HIV infection [9–13]. On the other hand, significant number of MCD patients are not infected with HHV-8 or HIV [10]. The term idiopathic MCD (iMCD) has been proposed for the latter cases based on an international evidence-based consensus diagnostic criteria [14].

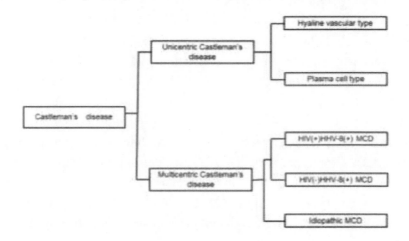

Figure 1. Classification of Castleman's disease. Castleman's disease is separated into multicentric Castleman's disease and unicentric Castleman's disease according to the number of affected lymph nodes. Furthermore, unicentric Castlaman's disease is pathologically divided into hyaline vascular and plasma cell types, and multicentric Castlaman's disease is classified based on HIV and HHV-8 status.

Table 1. MCD and similar disorders

Neoplastic	Inflammatory
Malignant lymphoma	Autoimmune disease
TAFRO syndrome	Adult-onset Still's disease
POEMS syndrome	Sjögren syndrome
IgG4-related disease	Rheumatoid arthritis
IPL	
ALPS	

MCD, Multicentric Castlman's Disease; TAFRO, Thrombocytopenia (T), Ascites (A), Fever (F), Reticulin Fibrosis in bone marrow (R), and Organomegaly (O); POEMS, polyneuropathy (P), organomegary (O), endocrinopathy (E), monoclonal gammopathy (M), and skin changes (S); IgG4, Immunoglobulin G4; IPL, Idiopathic plasmacytic lymphadenopathy; ALPS, autoimmune lymphoproliferative syndrome.

1.3. Idiopathic Multicentric Castleman's Disease (iMCD)

As with HHV-8-associated MCD, iMCD is also characterized by systemic inflammatory symptoms, which are triggered by proinflammatory hypercytokinemia [7]. Interleukin (IL)-6, vascular endothelial growth factor (VEGF), IL-1, and tumor necrosis factor (TNF)-α are thought to play significant roles in the pathogenesis of iMCD and HHV-8-associated MCD [15, 16]. Germinal centers of hyperplastic lymph nodes of patients with Castleman's disease produce large quantities of IL-6 [17] and the efficacy of anti-IL-6 therapy has been proven to improve the symptoms and biochemical abnormalities in MCD patients [18].

Although current literature suggests that IL-6 plays a critical role in MCD, the etiology of iMCD remains unclear. A variety of inflammatory responses are involved in the etiology of iMCD [15]. A considerable number of disorders such as infection-related disorders, autoimmune/ autoinflammatory diseases and malignant/lymphoproliferative disorders have similar clinicopathological characteristics as MCD, and recent international evidence-based consensus diagnostic criteria states the requirement of the exclusion of these disorders to make a diagnosis of iMCD [11]. A deep understanding of the similar disorders and a careful evaluation are necessary for accurate diagnosis.

1.4. TAFRO Syndrome

TAFRO syndrome was proposed by Takai et al. who reported three Japanese cases in 2010. TAFRO shares a constellation of clinical symptoms: thrombocytopenia (T), ascites (A), fever (F), reticulin fibrosis in bone marrow (R), and organomegaly (O) [19]. Although γ-globulin levels are not elevated in TAFRO syndrome, the histopathological findings of the lymph nodes of reported cases reveal a hyaline-vascular type consistent with MCD. Since the first description of TAFRO syndrome in Japan, cases have been described in Europe and the U.S., leading to the recognition of TAFRO syndrome as a subtype of MCD [20]. The pathogenesis of TAFRO syndrome has not been clarified: however, accumulating evidence suggests that it is an immunological disorder induced by a cytokine storm (hypercytokinemia), in which IL-6 and VEGF play critical roles, as found in other cases of MCD

[21, 22]. The diagnostic criteria for TAFRO-iMCD was proposed by Iwaki et al. (Table 2) [20].

Table 2. Diagnostic criteria for TAFRO-iMCD

1. Histopathological criteria;
Compatible with pathological findings of lymph nodes as TAFRO-iMCD[a]
Negative LANA-1 for HHV-8
2. Major criteria;
Presents 3 of 5 TAFRO symptoms
Thrombocytopenia
Anasarca
Fever
Reticulin fibrosis
Organomegaly
Absence of hypergammaglobulinemia
Small volume lymphadenopathy
3. Minor criteria need 1 or more;
Hyper/normoplasia of megakaryocytes in bone marrow
High levels of serum ALP without markedly elevated serum Transaminase

Requirements; fulfill histopathological criteria, all major criteria, and 1 or more of minor criteria. Diseases that should be excluded include rheumatologic diseases such as SLE, infectious diseases such as acute Epstein-Barr virus, and neoplastic diseases such as lymphoma, POEMS syndrome, and other cancers. a: TAFRO characteristic findings of lymph node, i.e., atrophic germinal centers with enlarged nuclei of endothelial cells, proliferation of endothelial venules with enlarged nuclear in interfollicular zone, and small numbers of mature plasma cells. iMCD: idiopathic multicentric Castleman's disease, LANA-1: latency-associated nuclear antigen 1, HHV-8: human herpes virus-8, ALP, alkaline phosphatase.

1.5. POEMS Syndrome

POEMS syndrome is a paraneoplastic syndrome caused by an underlying plasma cell neoplasm, which is characterized by polyneuropathy (P), organomegary (O), endocrinopathy (E), monoclonal gammopathy (M), and skin changes (S). Table 3 shows the diagnostic criteria of POEMS syndrome [23]. Overproduction of the cytokine VEGF is thought to be involved in the pathogenesis of POEMS syndrome. Typically, POEMS syndrome can be distinguished from CD by the presence of polyneuropathy and monoclonal plasma cells [24]. In addition, the cytokine IL-6 is more overexpressed in CD. However, some patients do not have both peripheral neuropathy and a plasma cell clone, and these patients are classified as having a CD variant of POEMS if they have other POEMS features [24]. POEMS syndrome is differentiated from MCD by the presence of monoclonal cells, and this is included in the exclusion criteria in the recent international evidence-based consensus diagnostic criteria for iMCD [14]. However, the difference between POEMS syndrome, especially the CD variant of POEMS, and MCD remains unclear.

Table 3. Diagnostic criteria of POEMS syndrome

Mandatory major criteria
1. Polyneuropathy (typically demyelinating)
2. Monoclonal plasma cell-proliferative disorder (almost always)
Other major criteria (one required)
3. CD
4. Sclerotic bone lesions
5. VEGF elevation
Minor criteria (one required)
6. Organomegaly (splenomegaly, hepatomegaly, or lymphadenopathy)
7. Extravascular volume overload (edema, pleural effusions, or ascites)
8. Endocrinopathy (adrenal, thyroid, pituitary, gonadal, parathyroid or pancreatic)
Minor criteria (one required)
9. Skin changes (hyperpigmentation, hypertrichosis, glomeruloid hemangiomata, plethora, acrocyanosis, flushing or white nails)
10. Papilledema
11. Thrombocytosis/polycythemia
Other symptoms and signs
Clubbing, weight loss, hyperhidrosis, pulmonary hypertension/restrictive lung disease, thrombotic diatheses, diarrhea, low vitamin B12 values

POEMS: polyneuropathy (P), organomegary (O), endocrinopathy (E), monoclonal gammopathy (M), and skin changes (S); CD: Castleman's disease; VEGF: vascular endothelial growth factor.

1.6. Immunoglobulin G4 (IgG4)-Related Disease

IgG4-related disease (IgG4-RD) is a recently described systemic fibroinflammatory disease [25]. It is associated with elevated serum IgG4 concentrations and infiltration by IgG4-positive plasma cells. Multifocal lymphadenopathy is often present, as well as MCD-like features [25]. IgG4-RD is sometimes difficult to distinguish from MCD due to the overlapping clinical characteristics, and lymph node lesions in IgG4-RD show histological and immunological findings similar to those observed in MCD [26, 27]. Lung lesions in IgG4-RD are characterized by active fibrosis with eosinophilic infiltration within the perilymphatic stromal area, and obstructive vasculitis [28]. In contrast, lung lesions in MCD are distinguished by lymphoplasmacyte proliferating lesions, which are mainly found in the alveolar area adjacent to the perilymphatic stromal region. Typically, histological characteristics and serum IL-6 levels may be helpful in differentiating MCD from IgG4-RD [28]. However, to distinguish between the two is sometimes difficult. Furthermore, some cases in which IgG4-RD and MCD are possibly overlapped are even reported [29, 30].

1.7. Autoimmune Diseases

Clinical features, such as rash, arthralgia, and neuropathy, are sometimes found in patients with MCD. The histological findings of lymphadenopathy in patients with connective tissue diseases (CTDs) are sometimes consistent with CD findings. According to one study, 29% (6/21) of patients with systemic lupus erythematosus had histological features of CD [31]. Kojima et al. reported seven cases of MCD combined with autoimmune disease, such as Sjögren syndrome or systemic sclerosis [32]. Lymphadenopathy is frequently found in cases of rheumatoid arthritis and sometimes resembles that observed in MCD [33]. CD may occur concomitantly, precede, or follow CTDs. Thus, it is often difficult to differentiate between CD and CTDs. Other autoimmune diseases, such as paraneoplastic pemphigus [34], and Evan's syndrome [35], have also been reported in patients with CD [36]. Thus, the complications of these autoimmune diseases should be carefully evaluated in such patients [37].

1.8. Idiopathic Plasmacytic Lymphadenopathy with Polyclonal Hypergammaglobulinemia (IPL)

IPL was first described as a new clinicopathological entity in 1980, and is considered identical to MCD in Western countries [38, 39]. Like MCD, IPL is characterized by multicentric lymphadenopathy, prominent hypergammaglobulinemia, and elevated serum IL-6 levels. However, based on a study of Japanese patients with MCD, Kojima et al. divided MCD into the IPL and non-IPL types [40]. They showed that the IPL type was characterized by male predominance, prominent polyclonal hyperimmunoglobulinemia and the histological plasma cell type. In contrast, female predominance, high incidence of pleural effusion or ascites, frequent association with autoimmune disease and the histological hyaline vascular or mixed type, were found in the non-IPL type. In addition, histological findings showed that the germinal centers of the IPL type tended to be normal in contrast to those of the non-IPL type, which can show various types such as normal, hyaline vascular and epithelioid types. Furthermore, the non-IPL type exhibited an aggressive and usually fatal disease course compared to the IPL type [39, 41]. However, these differences between the IPL and the non-IPL types have not been generally recognized yet. The recent international consensus diagnostic criteria temporally included IPL into iMCD [11].

1.9. Autoimmune Lymphoproliferative Syndrome (ALPS)

ALPS is a rare nonmalignant lymphoproliferative disorder, which is associated with increased $CD3^+$ T cell receptor (TCR) $\alpha\beta^+CD4^-CD8^-$ DNT cells and impaired lymphocyte apoptosis due to defects in the CD95 signaling cascade [42, 43]. Unregulated lymphocyte proliferation caused by impaired T-cell apoptosis results in lymphadenopathy, splenomegaly, and autoimmune cytopenia, all of which are typical in the clinical presentation of ALPS [41]. The diagnostic criteria for ALPS was created by consensus in 1999 and revised in 2010 by a group of international investigators. Table 4 provides a summary of the latest diagnostic criteria for ALPS [44]. Although the majority of ALPS patients have mutations in lymphocyte apoptosis-related genes, such as Fas, mutations in NRAS, KRAS, and caspase 8 are also associated with ALPS-like disorders [45–48]. However, genetic defects are undefined in some ALPS patients who meet the diagnostic criteria of ALPS [42]. As ALPS is a syndrome with variable phenotypes, which can overlap with other disorders, the differential diagnosis must distinguish it from various conditions, such as Evans' syndrome, hemophagocytic lymphohistiocytosis, and other lymphoproliferative disorders [42].

Table 4. Diagnostic criteria for ALPS

Required
1. Chronic (> 6 months), nonmalignant, noninfectious lymphadenopathy or splenomegaly or both
2. Elevated $CD3^+TCR\alpha\beta^+CD4^-CD8^-$ DNT cells ($\geq$ 1.5% of total lymphocytes or 2.5% of $CD3^+$ lymphocytes) in the setting of normal or elevated lymphocyte counts
Accessory
Primary
1. Defective lymphocyte apoptosis (in two separate assays)
2. Somatic or germline pathogenic mutation in FAS, FASLG, or CASP10
Secondary
1. Elevated plasma sFASL levels (> 200 pg/mL) OR elevated plasma IL-10 levels (> 20 pg/mL) OR elevated serum or plasma vitamin B12 levels (> 1500 ng/L) OR elevated plasma IL-18 levels > 500 pg/mL
2. Typical immunohistological findings as reviewed by an experienced hematopathologist
3. Autoimmune cytopenia (hemolytic anemia, thrombocytopenia, or neutropenia) AND elevated immunoglobulin G levels (polyclonal hypergammaglobulinemia)
4. Family history of nonmalignant/noninfectious lymphoproliferation, with or without autoimmunity

A definitive diagnosis is based on the presence of both the required criteria, in addition to one primary criterion. A probable diagnosis is based on the presence of both required criteria plus one secondary criterion. ALPS: autoimmune lymphoproliferative syndrome, TCR: T cell receptor: DNT: double-negative T cells, IL-10: interleukin-10, IL-18: interleukin-18, FASLG: Fas-ligand, CASP10: Caspase 10, sFASL: soluble FAS ligand.

2. PATHOGENESIS OF MCD

Previous reports demonstrated the involvement of HHV-8, which is recognized as one of the causes of CD, in the pathogenesis of MCD in HHV-8 positive MCD [15, 16]. In MCD, increases in several cytokines, such as IL-1, IL-6, IL-10, and TNF-α (i.e., hypercytokinemia), result in the presentation of clinical features, including fever, weight loss, and night sweats. IL-6, which is produced by B cells, monocytes, endothelial cells, and fibroblasts, modulates the acute phase response and resistance of T cells to apoptosis [17]. It also induces the activation of VEGF and T-helper cells, and the differentiation of B cells to plasma cells [15]. Yoshizaki et al. reported that IL-6 was produced in germinal centers of hyperplastic lymph nodes, and resection of the affected lymph nodes caused a clinical improvement and decrease in serum IL-6 levels in CD [17]. The results of studies have demonstrated the significance of IL-6 in the pathogenesis of CD [18].

HHV-8 replicates in germinal centers and infiltrating plasmablasts expressing viral IL-6 (vIL-6), and is reported to induce endogenous human IL-6 (hIL-6) in HHV-8-positive MCD [6, 49]. In HHV-8-negative MCD, some studies reported cytogenetic abnormalities or prevalent gene polymorphisms that involved in IL-6 or IL-6 receptor genes [50]. Beneficial effects of IL-6 signaling blockage have been shown in patients with MCD, although the precise mechanisms of elevated IL-6 levels are unclear [18]. The clinical features of HHV-8 negative MCD depend on the type of disorder or combination of disorders (i.e., neoplastic, inflammatory, or infectious) [15, 20]. Gakipoulou et al. reported a case of MCD complicated by Evan's syndrome, suggesting that an autoimmune mechanism may also be involved in the pathogenesis of MCD [35]. A case of Epstein-Barr (EB) virus infection complicated by MCD was also reported [48]. These reports suggest that HHV-8 negative MCD includes a variety of disorders. Fajgenbaum et al. proposed diagnostic criteria of iMCD that requires careful evaluation in order to make an accurate diagnosis based on the clinical presentation, additional biopsies, serologic or microbiology studies, and careful clinical correlation [11].

There is little evidence showing a relationship between ALPS and MCD. To the best of our knowledge, our recently published case is the sole report describing the possible relationship between ALPS and MCD [51]. Although ALPS is included in the exclusion criteria of iMCD [11], we need to debate about whether the diagnostic criteria of iMCD are reasonable. We present and discuss clinical characteristics of our MCD case with ALPS-like features in the next section.

3. PATIENT PRESENTATION

We recently described a case of MCD with ALPS-like features [51]. The patient was a 37-year old woman who presented with fatigue, dyspnea, and a slight fever. She had a history of type-I diabetes and Grave's disease. Chest radiographs and computed tomography revealed diffuse ground grass opacities, small nodules in both lung fields, and hilar and mediastinal lymphadenopathy. Histopathological findings of the lung and mediastinal lymph node biopsy showed infiltration of polyclonal and plasma cells, which were consistent with the plasma cell type of CD. In addition, both plasma IL-6 and VEGF levels were elevated. A diagnosis of MCD was made. The percentage of DNT cells (4.9% of total T cells) exceeded the criterion for ALPS (Table 4). Fas-induced apoptosis of lymphocytes was also impaired [44]. Although the diagnostic criteria for ALPS requires to show a mutation in FAS, FASLG, or CASP10 or lymphocyte apoptosis in two separate assays, it was unfortunate that we performed just one assay to show the impairment of Fas-induced lymphocyte apoptosis. However, we considered that our patient had ALPS based on a careful evaluation of the clinicopathological findings. Following treatment with oral corticosteroids, both pulmonary infiltration and anemia improved.

4. SIMILARITY OF CLINICOPATHOLOGICAL FEATURES OF MCD AND ALPS

Lymphadenopathy, autoimmunity, and clinicopathological pulmonary involvement are common manifestations of both MCD and ALPS. ALPS is linked to the development of multiple autoimmune disorders [52]. Pulmonary involvement (parenchymal lung disease) is a characteristic of both MCD and ALPS. Computed tomography findings of pulmonary involvement in ALPS are ground-glass opacities, large nodules, tree-in bud nodules, bronchiectasis, and septal thickening [53]. In MCD, diffuse centrilobular pulmonary parenchymal nodular opacities and ground-glass opacities are the major radiological findings [54, 55], indicating the similarity of radiological findings between MCD and ALPS.

Fas/Fas ligand-deficient *lpr* and *gld* mice show an increase in DNT cells, autoimmunity, and lymphoproliferation, with massive and systemic enlargement of lymph nodes [56]. In histological evaluations of lymph nodes of ALPS patients, a prominent reactive germinal center, as well as lymphocytic proliferation of histiocytes and plasma cells, are commonly observed [53]. Reactive follicular hyperplasia, often with focal progressive transformation of the germinal center and polyclonal plasmacytosis, is an additional histological feature of enlarged lymph nodes in ALPS [53, 57]. These pathological findings of lymph nodes in ALPS are compatible with those in MCD. However, the clinicopathological findings of ALPS and MCD have not been compared in detail.

4.1. CD4 and CD8 Double-Negative T (DNT) Cells

An increase in DNT cells is one of the characteristic features of ALPS. Lymphocyte apoptosis plays an important role in sustaining lymphocyte homeostasis, peripheral immune tolerance and preventing autoimmunity, and is triggered by the activation of the cell surface receptor Fas [58]. Although defects in the intrinsic apoptotic pathway mediated by Fas is believed to be associated with the accumulation of DNT cells, recent research suggested a critical role for Bcl-2 family members and the intrinsic apoptotic pathway in controlling T-cell responses [59]. Thus, the roles of extrinsic and intrinsic apoptotic pathways may overlap in T-cell homeostasis [60]. Overall, an increase in DNT cells and functional defects in T cells in an *in vitro* FAS-induced apoptosis assay are helpful in the diagnosis of ALPS [61]. On the other hand, to the best of our knowledge, our case is the sole published report describing the possible relationship between ALPS and MCD [51]. To date, there has been little evidence showing the relationship between ALPS and MCD. In this regard, it is better to include ALPS with MCD-like features into iMCD at this time, although the recent international consensus diagnostic criteria excludes ALPS from iMCD [11].

CONCLUSION

The precise etiology of MCD remains unclear, and various diseases can present MCD-like features. Although the international diagnostic criteria haves been proposed for iMCD, caution is needed in its application. Some disorders (e.g., ALPS) have been included in the exclusion criteria without full clarification of the relationship between MCD and these disorders. A definite diagnosis of MCD should be made with careful evaluation, especially in HHV-8 negative cases. Further investigations are necessary to understand the pathophysiology of MCD and its relationship with other related disorders. Observations of more MCD cases with ALPS or ALPS-like features can shed light on the relationship between these rare lymphoproliferative disorders.

DISCLOSURE

The authors declare no conflict of interests. Funding: None.

REFERENCES

[1] Castleman, B., Iverson, L., Menendez, V. P. (1956). Localized mediastinal lymph node hyperplasia resembling thymoma. *Cancer*, 9(4): 822-830.

[2] Wang, H. W., Pittaluga, S., Jaffe, E. S. (2016). Multicentric Castleman disease: Where are we now? *Semin Diagn Pathol*, 33(5): 294-306.

[3] Harris. N. L. (1984). Hypervascular follicular hyperplasia and Kaposi's sarcoma in patients at risk for AIDS. *New Engl J Med*, 310(7): 462-463.

[4] Lachant, N. A., Sun, N. C., Leong, L. A., Oseas, R. S., and Prince, H. E. (1985). Multicentric angiofollicular lymph node hyperplasia (Castleman's disease) followed by Kaposi's sarcoma in two homosexual males with the acquired immunodeficiency syndrome (AIDS). *Am J Clin Pathol*, 83(1): 27-33.

[5] Keller, A. R., Hochholzer, L., and Castleman, B. (1972). Hyaline-vascular and plasma-cell types of giant lymph node hyperplasia of the mediastinum and other locations. *Cancer*, 29(3): 670-683.

[6] Dossier, A., Meignin, V., Fieschi, C., Boutboul, D., Oksenhendler, E., and Galicier, L. (2013). Human herpesvirus 8-related Castleman disease in the absence of HIV infection. *Clin Infect Dis*, 56(6): 833-842.

[7] Liu, A. Y., Nabel, C. S., Finkelman, B. S., Ruth, J. R., Kurzrock, R., van Rhee, F., Krymskaya, V. P., Kelleher, D., Rubenstein, A. H., and Fajgenbaum, D. C. (2016). Idiopathic multicentric Castleman's disease: a systematic literature review. *Lancet Haematol*, 3(4): e163-175.

[8] Dupin, N., Fisher, C., Kellam, P., Ariad, S., Tulliez, M., Franck, N., van Marck, E., Salmon, D., Gorin, I., Escande, J. P., Weiss, R. A., Alitalo, K., and Boshoff, C. (1999). Distribution of human herpesvirus-8 latently infected cells in Kaposi's sarcoma, multicentric Castleman's disease, and primary effusion lymphoma. *Proc Natl Acad Sci U S A*, 96(8): 4546-4551.

[9] Soulier, J., Grollet, L., Oksenhendler, E., Cacoub, P., Cazals-Hatem, D., Babinet, P., d'Agay, M. F., Clauvel, J. P., Raphael, M., Degos, L., and Sigaux, F. (1995). Kaposi's sarcoma-associated herpesvirus-like DNA sequences in multicentric Castleman's disease. *Blood*, 86(4): 1276-1280.

[10] Barozzi, P., Luppi, M., Masini, L., Marasca, R., Savarino, M., Morselli, M., Ferrari, M. G., Bevini, M., Bonacorsi, G., and Torelli, G. (1996). Lymphotropic herpes virus (EBV, HHV-6, HHV-8) DNA sequences in HIV negative Castleman's disease. *Clin Mol Pathol*, 49(4): M232-235.

[11] Dupin, N., Diss, T. L., Kellam, P., Tulliez, M., Du, M. Q., Sicard, D., Weiss, R. A., Isaacson, P. G., and Boshoff, C. (2000). HHV-8 is associated with a plasmablastic variant of Castleman disease that is linked to HHV-8-positive plasmablastic lymphoma. *Blood*, 95(4): 1406-1412.

[12] Chang, Y., Cesarman, E., Pessin, M. S., Lee, F., Culpepper, J., Knowles, D. M., and Moore, P. S. (1994). Identification of herpesvirus-like DNA sequences in AIDS-associated Kaposi's sarcoma. *Science*, 266(5192): 1865-1869.

[13] Moore, P. S., Boshoff, C., Weiss, R. A., and Chang, Y. (1996). Molecular mimicry of human cytokine and cytokine response pathway genes by KSHV. *Science*, 274(5293): 1739-1744.

[14] Fajgenbaum, D. C., Uldrick, T. S., Bagg, A., Frank, D., Wu, D., Srkalovic, G., Simpson, D., Liu, A. Y., Menke, D., Chandrakasan, S., Lechowicz, M. J., Wong, R. S., Pierso,n S., Paessler, M., Rossi, J. F., Ide, M., Ruth. J., Croglio, M., Suarez, A., Krymskaya, V., Chadburn, A., Colleoni, G., Nasta, S., Jayanthan, R., Nabel, C. S., Casper, C., Dispenzieri, A., Fosså, A., Kelleher, D., Kurzrock, R., Voorhees, P., Dogan, A., Yoshizaki, K., van Rhee, F., Oksenhendler, E., Jaffe, E. S., Elenitoba-Johnson, K. S., and Lim, M. S. (2017). International, evidence-based consensus diagnostic criteria for HHV-8-negative/idiopathic multicentric Castleman disease. *Blood*, 129(12): 1646-1657.

[15] Fajgenbaum, D. C., van Rhee, F., and Nabel, C. S. (2014). HHV-8-negative, idiopathic multicentric Castleman disease: novel insights into biology, pathogenesis, and therapy. *Blood*, 123(19): 2924-2933.
[16] van Rhee, F., Stone, K., Szmania, S., Barlogie, B., and Singh, Z. (2010). Castleman disease in the 21st century: an update on diagnosis, assessment, and therapy. *Clin Adv Hematol Oncol*, 8(7): 486-498.
[17] Yoshizaki, K., Matsuda, T., Nishimoto, N., Kuritani, T., Taeho, L., Aozasa, K., Nakahata, T., Kawai, H., Tagoh, H., and Komori, T. (1989). Pathogenic significance of interleukin-6 (IL-6/BSF-2) in Castleman's disease. *Blood*, 74(4): 1360-1367.
[18] Nishimoto, N., Kanakura, Y., Aozasa, K., Johkoh, T., Nakamura, M., Nakano, S., Nakano, N., Ikeda, Y., Sasaki, T., Nishioka, K., Hara, M., Taguchi, H., Kimura, Y., Kato, Y., Asaoku, H., Kumagai, S., Kodama, F., Nakahara, H., Hagihara, K., Yoshizaki, K., and Kishimoto, T. (2005). Humanized anti-interleukin-6 receptor antibody treatment of multicentric Castleman disease. *Blood*, 106(8): 2627-2632.
[19] Srkalovic, G., Marijanovic, I., Srkalovic, M. B., and Fajgenbaum. D. C. (2017) TAFRO syndrome: New subtype of idiopathic multicentric Castleman disease. *Bosn J Basic Med Sci,* 17(2), 81-84.
[20] Iwaki, N., Fajgenbaum, D. C., Nabel, C. S., Gion, Y., Kondo, E., Kawano, M., Masunari, T., Yoshida, I., Moro, H., Nikkuni, K., Takai, K., Matsue, K., Kurosama, M., Hagihara, M., Saito, A., Okamoto, M., Yokota, K., Hiraiwa, S., Nakamura, N., Nakao, S., Yoshino, T., and Sato, Y. (2016). Clinicopathologic analysis of TAFRO syndrome demonstrates a distinct subtype of HHV-8-negative multicentric Castleman disease. *Am J Hematol*, 91(2): 220-226.
[21] Carbone, A., and Pantanowitz, L. (2016). TAFRO syndrome: An atypical variant of KSHV-negative multicentric Castleman disease. *Am J Hematol*, 91(2): 171-172.
[22] Kubokawa, I., Yachie, A., Hayakawa, A., Hirase, S., Yamamoto, N., Mori, T., Yanai, T., Takeshima, Y., Kyo, E., Kageyama, G., Nagai, H., Uehara, K., Kojima, M., and Iijima, K. (2014). The first report of adolescent TAFRO syndrome, a unique clinicopathologic variant of multicentric Castleman's disease. *BMC Pediatr*, 14:139.

[23] Dispenzieri, A. POEMS syndrome: 2014 update on diagnosis, risk-stratification, and management. (2014). *Am J Hematol*, 89(2): 214-223.
[24] Dispenzieri, A. POEMS syndrome: update on diagnosis, risk-stratification, and management. (2015). *Am J Hematol*, 90(10): 951-962.
[25] Cheuk, W., and Chan, J. K. (2012). Lymphadenopathy of IgG4-related disease: an underdiagnosed and overdiagnosed entity. *Semin Diagn Pathol*, 29(4): 226-234.
[26] Zoshima T, Yamada K, Hara S, Mizushima, I., Yamagishi, M., Harada, K., Sato, Y., and Kawano, M. (2016). Multicentric Castleman disease with tubulointerstitial nephritis mimicking IgG4-related disease: two case reports. *Am J Surg Pathol*, 40(4): 495-501.
[27] Ikeura, T., Horitani, S., Masuda, M., Kasai, T., Yanagawa, M., Miyoshi, H., Uchida, K., Takaoka, M., Miyasaka, C., Uemura, Y., and Okazaki, K. (2016). IgG4-related Disease Involving Multiple Organs with Elevated Serum Interleukin-6 Levels. *Intern Med*, 55(18): 2623-2628.
[28] Terasaki, Y., Ikushima, S., Matsui, S., Hebisawa, A., Ichimura, Y., Izumi, S., Ujita, M., Arita, M., Tomii, K., Komase, Y., Owan, I., Kawamura, T., Matsuzawa, Y., Murakami, M., Ishimoto, H., Kimura, H., Bando, M., Nishimoto, N., Kawabata, Y., Fukuda. Y., and Ogura, T.; Tokyo Diffuse Lung Diseases Study Groupe. (2017). Comparison of clinical and pathological features of lung lesions of systemic IgG4-related disease and idiopathic multicentric Castleman's disease. *Histopathology*, 70(7): 1114-1124.
[29] Terasaki, Y., Ikushima, S., Matsui, S., Ogoshi, T., Kido, T., Yatera, K., Oda, K., Kawanami, T., Ishimoto, H., Sakamoto, N., Sano, A., Yoshii, C., Shimajiri, S., and Mukae, H. (2013). Assessment of pathologically diagnosed patients with Castleman's disease associated with diffuse parenchymal lung involvement using the diagnostic criteria for IgG4-related disease. *Lung*, 191(6): 575-583.
[30] Ikari, J., Kojima, M., Tomita, K., Nakamura, T., Toyoda, F., Otsuki, Y., Shimizu, S., Kobayashi, H., and Nakamura, H. (2010). A case of

IgG4-related lung disease associated with multicentric Castleman's disease and lung cancer. *Intern Med*, 49(13): 1287-1291.

[31] Kojima, M., Nakamura, S., Morishita, Y., Itoh, H., Yoshida, K., Ohno, Y., Oyama, T., Asano, S., Joshita, T., Mori, S., Suchi, T., and Masawa, N. (2000). Reactive follicular hyperplasia in the lymph node lesions from systemic lupus erythematosus patients: a clinicopathological and immunohistological study of 21 cases. *Pathol Int*, 50(4): 304-312.

[32] Kojima, M., Nakamura, N., Tsukamoto, N., Yokohama, A., Itoh, H., Kobayashi, S., Kashimura, M., Masawa, N., and Nakamura, S. (2011). Multicentric Castleman's disease representing effusion at initial clinical presentation: clinicopathological study of seven cases. *Lupus*, 20(1): 44-50.

[33] Kojima, M., Motoori, T., and Nakamura, S. (2006). Benign, atypical and malignant lymphoproliferative disorders in rheumatoid arthritis patients. *Biomed Pharmacother*, 60(10): 663-672.

[34] Nikolskaia, O. V., Nousari, C. H., and Anhalt, G. J. (2003). Paraneoplastic pemphigus in association with Castleman's disease. *Br J Dermatol*, 149(6): 1143-1151.

[35] Gakiopoulou, H., Korkolopoulou, P., Paraskevakou, H., Marinaki, S., Voulgarelis, M., Stofas, A., Lelouda, M., Lazaris, A. C., Boletis, J., and Patsouris, E. (2010). Membranoproliferative glomerulonephritis in the setting of multicentric angiofollicular lymph node hyperplasia (Castleman's disease) complicated by Evan's syndrome. *J Clin Pathol*, 63(6): 552-554.

[36] De Marchi, G., De Vita, S., Fabris, M., Scott, C. A., and Ferraccioli, G. (2004). Systemic connective tissue disease complicated by Castleman's disease: report of a case and review of the literature. *Haematologica*, 89(4): ECR03.

[37] Muskardin, T. W., Peterson, B. A., and Molitor, J. A. (2012). Castleman disease and associated autoimmune disease. *Curr Opin Rheumatol*, 24(1): 76-83.

[38] Frizzera, G. (1988). Castleman's disease and related disorders. *Semin Deagn Pathol*, 5(4): 346-364.

[39] Frizzera, G. (2000). Atypical lymphoproliferative disorders. In Knowles, D. M., (Ed), *Neoplastic Hematopathology*. (2nd ed, pp. 569-622). Baltimore, USA: Lippincott Williams & Wilkins.
[40] Kojima, M., Nakamura, N., Tsukamoto, N., Otuski, Y., Shimizu, K., Itoh, H., Kobayashi, S., Kobayashi, H., Murase, T., Masawa, N., Kashimura, M., and Nakamura, S. (2008). Clinical implications of idiopathic multicentric Castleman disease among Japanese: a report of 28 cases. *Int J Surg Patho*l, 16(4): 391-398.
[41] Kojima, M., Nakamura, S., Shimizu, K., Itoh, H., Yamane, Y., Murayama, K., Tanaka, H., Sugihara, S., Shimano, S., Sakata, N., and Masawa, N. (2004). Clinical implication of idiopathic plasmacytic lymphadenopathy with polyclonal hypergamma-globulinemia: a report of 16 cases. *Int J Surg Pathol*, 12(1): 25-30.
[42] Shah, S., Wu, E., Rao, V. K., Tarrant, T. K. (2014). Autoimmune lymphoproliferative syndrome: an update and review of the literature. *Curr Allergy Asthma Rep*, 14(9): 462.
[43] Fisher, G. H., Rosenberg, F. J., Straus, S.E., Dale, J. K., Middleton, L. A., Lin, A. Y., Strober, W., Lenardo, M. J., and Puck, J. M. (1995). Dominant interfering Fas gene mutations impair apoptosis in a human autoimmune lymphoproliferative syndrome. *Cell*, 81(6): 935-946.
[44] Oliveira, J. B., Bleesing, J. J., Dianzani, U., Fleisher, T. A., Jaffe, E. S., Lenardo, M. J., Rieux-Laucat, F., Siegel, R. M., Su, H. C., Teachey, D. T., and Rao, V. K. (2010). Revised diagnostic criteria and classification for the autoimmune lymphoproliferative syndrome (ALPS): report from the 2009 NIH International Workshop. *Blood*, 116(14): e35-40.
[45] Oliveira, J. B., Bidere, N., Niemela, J. E., Zheng, L., Sakai, K., Nix, C. P., Danner, R. L., Barb, J., Munson, P. J., Puck, J. M., Dale, J., Straus, S. E., Fleisher, T. A., and Lenardo, M. J. (2007). NRAS mutation causes a human autoimmune lymphoproliferative syndrome. *Proc Natl Acad Sci U S A*, 104(21): 8953-8958.

[46] Takagi, M., Shinoda, K., Piao, J., Mitsuiki, N., Takagi, M., Matsuda, K., Muramatsu, H., Doisaki, S., Nagasawa, M., Morio, T., Kasahara, Y., Koike, K., Kojima, S., Takao, A., and Mizutani, S. (2011). Autoimmune lymphoproliferative syndrome-like disease with somatic KRAS mutation. *Blood*, 117(10): 2887-2890.
[47] Bidere, N., Su, H. C., and Lenardo, M. J. (2006). Genetic disorders of programmed cell death in the immune system. *Annu Rev Immunol*, 24:321-52.
[48] Salmena, L., and Hakem, R. (2005). Caspase-8 deficiency in T cells leads to a lethal lymphoinfiltrative immune disorder. *J Exp Med*, 202(6): 727-732.
[49] Mori, Y., Nishimoto, N., Ohno, M., Inagi, R., Dhepakson, P., Amou, K., Yoshizaki, K., and Yamanishi, K. (2000). Human herpesvirus 8-encoded interleukin-6 homologue (viral IL-6) induces endogenous human IL-6 secretion. *J Med Virol*, 61(3): 332-335.
[50] Stone, K., Woods, E., Szmania, S. M., Stephens, O. W., Garg, T. K., Barlogie, B., Shaughnessy, J. D. Jr., Hall, B., Reddy, M., Hoering, A., Hansen, E., and van Rhee, F. (2013). Interleukin-6 receptor polymorphism is prevalent in HIV-negative Castleman Disease and is associated with increased soluble interleukin-6 receptor levels. *PLoS One,* 8(1): e54610.
[51] Minemura, H., Ikeda, K., Tanino, Y., Hashimoto, Y., Nikaido, T., Fukuhara, A., Yokouchi, H., Sato, S., Tanino, M., Oka, T., Hebisawa, A., Suzuki, H., Ogawa, K., Takeishi, Y., and Munakata, M. (2015). Multicentric Castleman's disease with impaired lymphocytic apoptosis. *Allergol Int*, 64(1): 112-114.
[52] Neven, B., Magerus-Chatinet, A., Florkin, B., Gobert, D., Lambotte, O., De Somer, L., Lanzarotti, N., Stolzenberg, M. C., Bader-Meunier, B., Aladjidi, N., Chantrain, C., Bertrand, Y., Jeziorski, E., Leverger, G., Michel, G., Suarez, F., Oksenhendler, E., Hermine, O., Blanche, S., Picard, C., Fischer, A., and Rieux-Laucat, F. (2011). A survey of 90 patients with autoimmune lymphoproliferative syndrome related to TNFRSF6 mutation. *Blood*, 118(18): 4798-4807.

[53] Lau, C. Y., Mihalek, A. D., Wang, J., Dodd, L. E., Perkins, K., Price, S., Webster, S., Pittaluga, S., Folio, L. R., Rao, V. K., and Olivier, K. N. (2016). Pulmonary Manifestations of the Autoimmune Lymphoproliferative Syndrome. A Retrospective Study of a Unique Patient Cohort. *Ann Am Thorac Soc*, 13(8): 1279-1288.

[54] Johkoh, T., Muller, N. L., Ichikado, K., Nishimoto, N., Yoshizaki, K., Honda, O., Tomiyama, N., Naitoh, H., Nakamura, H., and Yamamoto, S. (1998). Intrathoracic multicentric Castleman disease: CT findings in 12 patients. *Radiology*, 209(2): 477-81.

[55] Bonekamp, D., Horton, K. M., Hruban, R. H., and Fishman, E. K. (2011). Castleman disease: the great mimic. *Radiographics*, 31(6): 1793-1807.

[56] Murphy, E., and Roths, J. (1978). Autoimmunity and lymphoproliferation: induction by mutant gene *lpr*, and acceleration by a male-associated factor in strain BXSB mice. In: Rose NR, Bigazzi PE, Warner NL (Eds), *Genetic Control of Autoimmune Disease.* (pp. 207-219). New York, USA: Elsevier North Holland.

[57] Lim, M. S., Straus, S. E., Dale, J. K., Fleisher, T. A., Stetler-Stevenson, M., Strober, W., Sneller, M. C., Puck, J. M., Lenardo, M. J., Elenitoba-Johnson, K. S., Lin, A. Y., Raffeld, M., and Jaffe, E. (1998). Pathological findings in human autoimmune lymphoproliferative syndrome. *Am J Pathol*, 153(5): 1541-1550.

[58] Siegel, R. M., Chan, F. K., Chun, H. J., and Lenardo, M. J. (2000). The multifaceted role of Fas signaling in immune cell homeostasis and autoimmunity. *Nat Immunol*, 1(6): 469-474.

[59] Kurtulus, S., Tripathi, P., and Hildeman, D. A. (2013). Protecting and rescuing the effectors: roles of differentiation and survival in the control of memory T cell development. *Front Immunol*, 3: 404.

[60] Niss, O., Sholl, A., Bleesing, J. J., and Hildeman, D. A. (2015). IL-10/Janus kinase/signal transducer and activator of transcription 3 signaling dysregulates Bim expression in autoimmune lymphoproliferative syndrome. *J Allergy Clin Immunol*, 135(3): 762-770.

[61] Magerus-Chatinet, A., Stolzenberg, M. C., Loffredo, M. S., Neven, B., Schaffner, C., Ducrot, N., Arkwright, P. D., Bader-Meunier, B., Barbot, J., Blanche, S., Casanova, J. L., Debré, M., Ferster, A., Fieschi, C., Florkin, B., Galambrun, C., Hermine, O., Lambotte, O., Solary, E., Thomas, C., Le Deist, F., Picard, C., Fischer, A., and Rieux-Laucat, F. (2009). FAS-L, IL-10, and double-negative CD4- CD8- TCR alpha/beta+ T cells are reliable markers of autoimmune lymphoproliferative syndrome (ALPS) associated with FAS loss of function. *Blood*, 113(13): 3027-3030.

In: Advances in Health and Disease
Editor: Lowell T. Duncan

ISBN: 978-1-53613-020-1
© 2018 Nova Science Publishers, Inc.

Chapter 7

INFLUENCE OF GUT MICROBIOTA ON INFLAMMATORY BOWEL DISEASE

Dennis Cesar Levano-Linares[1],*, MD,
Patricia Sanchez-Salcedo[2],
David Alias-Jimenez [1], MD, PhD,
Belen Manso-Abajo[1], MD,
Ana Moreno-Posada[1], MD
and Jaime Ruiz-Tovar[1], MD, PhD

[1]Department of Surgery, University Hospital Rey Juan Carlos, Mostoles, Madrid, Spain
[2]Department of Surgical Nursery, Fundacion Jimenez Diaz, Madrid, Spain

ABSTRACT

Inflammatory bowel disease (IBD) is a chronic, multifactorial immune disorder and it is classified in two different entities with unknown etiologies: Crohn's Disease and Ulcerative Colitis. However, it is believed

---

* Corresponding Author E-mail: cesdenlinares@gmail.com.

that disturbance of the immune system and/or imbalanced interactions with microbes (dysbioses) leads to development of chronic intestinal inflammation. Over the past decade, IBD have emerged as one of the most studied human conditions linked to the gut microbiota. More recently, profiling studies of the intestinal microbiome have associated pathogenesis of IBD with characteristic shifts in the composition of the intestinal microbiota, reinforcing the view that IBD result from altered interactions between intestinal microbes and the mucosal immune system. On the other hand, several pathogens have been proposed as causative microorganisms for IBD development. Several factors can intervene with microbial gut community composition, including genetics, diet, age, drug treatment or smoking. The importance of each of these factors is still unclear, but several of them are directly or indirectly linked to disease state. Some studies show that the gut microbiota is an essential factor in driving inflammation in IBD and indeed, short-term treatment with some antibiotics reduces intestinal inflammation.

The improvements to DNA sequencing technology have set the stage for investigations of the IBD microbiome. Many studies find dysbioses, that occur in IBD and a broad pattern has begun to emerge which includes a reduction in biodiversity, a decreased and an increased representation of several taxa. As opposed, several lines of evidence suggest that specific groups of gut bacteria may have protective effects against IBD. It is important to mention that some of the alterations observed in the colorectal cancer (CRC) microbiome are also observed in IBD, and chronic intestinal inflammation is a major risk factor for the development of CRC.

Despite promising correlations between microbial composition and disease phenotypes, to date no causative role for the microbiome has been established, and our understanding of the dynamic role of the human microbiome in IBD remains incomplete.

In this chapter, we will discuss the actual evidence about the involvement of microbiota on the appearance and development of IBD, and the eventual response to medical treatment.

Keywords: inflammatory bowel disease, Crohn's disease, ulcerative colitis, gut microbiota

INTRODUCTION

The term Inflammatory Bowel Disease (IBD) is applied generically to all chronic, multifactorial and idiopathic inflammatory processes, unlike other inflammatory diseases in which the etiological agent is known. Under this term two entities are included: Crohn's disease (CD) and Ulcerative colitis (UC), which together affect over 3.6 million people worldwide [1].

CD is a granulomatous and progressive transmural inflammation of gastrointestinal tract that can affect any part of the digestive tract, although the most frequently affected areas are the distal portions of small intestine (ileum) and the cecum. Its distribution is usually patchy and discontinuous. Extramural complications, such as abscesses or fistulas, are often associated.

UC is a recurrent and non-granulomatous chronic inflammatory disease, whose involvement is only limited to the colon mucosa. It affects only the colon and rectum, the distal location being more frequent, and the distribution is continuous with an ascending extension [2, 3].

In about 10% of cases with colonic involvement, a definitive diagnosis of CD or UC is not possible, thus the concept of Indeterminated Colitis is then raised [4].

Both pathologies include intestinal malabsorption, diarrhea, rectal bleeding, fever, abdominal pain and weight loss [5]. Both, CD and UC may present extraintestinal symptoms, which consist mainly of arthritis and low back pain, canker sores, cutaneous ulcers and liver disorders.

Epidemiology

The incidence of the disease has been on the rise over the past few decades, further highlighting the role of environmental factors in this disease.

In recent years, there has been a progressive increase in diagnosis in Western countries, with an incidence of 5.9/100,000 and 9.75/100,000 cases per year in CD in UC, respectively [6]. There is a greater incidence and prevalence in northern Europe and North America, while the lowest prevalence has been shown in continental Asia. The environment and lifestyle in developed countries, which is associated with smoking, high fat and sugar diets, drug use, stress and high socioeconomic status are linked to the occurrence of IBD and various metabolic disorders.

IBD has a first incidence peak between 15 and 30 years and a later peak between 50 and 70 years [1]. It is unclear whether this late-onset pick represents an increased incidence over the years, a late expression of early environmental exposure, or it is a misdiagnosis of an underlying vascular disease. Males and females have the same risk of developing IBD.

Numerous studies have shown that there is familial aggregation, with concordance rates in monozygotic twins of 10% in UC and 40-50% in CD [7]. In patients with a first-degree relative with IBD, the development risk is 8-15 folds and 20-30 folds higher than general population in UC and CD, respectively [8].

Etiopathogeny

Major advances have occurred in the knowledge of the pathogenesis of IBD. All clinical and experimental evidence suggest that BD is a multifactorial disorder that occur due to a complex interaction between the microbiome, the immune system and environmental factors in a genetically predisposed subject [9]. The increase in prevalence of IBD worldwide, particularly in socioeconomically evolving countries, shows a basis for an environmental influence on IBD development.

Age

An important environmental factor is age. There is an age-related variation in the distribution of IBD phenotypes, with three distinct stages of onset. A peak age of onset is typically between 15 and 30 years old, with late onset cases occurring in the 6th decade of life and early onset in childs younger than 10 years old. Noticeably, the latter group has shown a significant increase in incidence over the last decade [10]. These stages correspond to phases in which the gut microbiota alters its diversity and stability [11]. Early life is marked by a microbiome of low complexity and low stability; this microbiota is more volatile, affected by the birth route, and fluctuates with events, such as changes in diet (switch from breastfeeding to solid foods), illness, and puberty [12]. It takes until adulthood for the microbial assemblage to reach a maximal stability and complexity, with improved resilience towards perturbations [13]. However, decreased stability has been observed in the elderly (60 years or older) [14]. Given these different characteristics of the microbiome at the three distinct stages of disease onset, a different role for the microbiome in disease initiation and progression should be considered.

Diet

One of the most important environmental factors impacting microbial composition is dietary preference, which has been demonstrated to determine microbiome composition throughout mammalian evolution [15].

Although no specific diet has been shown to directly cause, prevent, or treat IBD, it is important to take interactions between nutrients and microbiota into account when studying the role of the microbiome in disease. Wu et al. have shown that long-term dietary patterns affect the ratios of *Bacteroides*, *Prevotella*, and *Firmicutes*, and that short-term changes may not have major influences [16]. In addition, Zimmer et al. have studied the impact of a strict vegan or vegetarian diet on the microbiota [17], and found a significant reduction in *Bacteroides* spp., *Bifidobacterium* spp., and the *Enterobacteriaceae*, while total bacterial load remain unaltered. Since the *Enterobacteriaceae* are among the taxa that are consistently found to be increased in patients with IBD, it would be valuable to include both short- and long-term dietary patterns in future studies of the role of the microbiome in IBD. Given the complexity of dietary effects, such information will only be feasible in a large cohort study [18].

Smoking

Cigarette smoking has a polarizing influence on the two main forms of IBD, whereby smoking is both a risk and aggravating influence on the CD, whereas in UC, the cessation of smoking is a risk factor for relapse and active smoking has a modest beneficial influence.

Acute Appendicitis

An episode of acute appendicitis, particularly in childhood or early adolescence, has a protective factor on the risk of developing UC.

Gut Microbiota

The intestinal microbial community is one of the factors that is gaining increasing attention, not only due to its influence on IBD, but also because of its role in many aspects of health [19]. The gut microbiota, the reservoir of microbes in the body, is recognized as an organ in its own [20] and coexists in equilibrium with its host in varying amounts throughout the gastrointestinal tract, reaching its greatest level in the colon with 10^{11} or 10^{12} cells/g of luminal contents [21].

Although some environmental and lifestyle factors, such as stress, drug therapy or pollution, might have independent influences on disease activity, most of the elements of a modern lifestyle in socioeconomically developed countries shape the composition and functional activity of the gut microbiota.

The microbiota assists in the degradation of otherwise indigestible carbohydrates in the human intestine through some digestive enzymes derived from bacteria [22]. Most nutrients produced by host enzymes are absorbed in the stomach and small intestine, whereas bacteria residing in the ileum usually utilize only simple carbohydrates as a major energy source [23]. By contrast, the indigestible carbohydrates and proteins equivalent to 10–30% of the total ingested energy reach the colon [24], where these otherwise indigestible dietary carbohydrates and host-derived glycans are converted by enzymes produced by strict anaerobic bacteria to simple carbohydrates used as nutrients and energy [25]. To do this, for instance, *Bacteroides* species possess many genes that encode essential enzymes to degrade diverse complex carbohydrates, and members of the phyla *Firmicutes*, *Actinobacteria* and *Verrucomicrobium* produce nutritionally specialized enzymes that have a key role in the degradation of substrates, such as plant cell walls, starch particles and mucins.

Also, anaerobic intestinal bacteria produce short-chain fatty acids (SCFAs) as the end products of fermentation of dietary fibers, among which, acetate, propionate and butyrate are the most abundant [26]. SCFAs are transported from the intestinal lumen into the various tissues where they are used as either a source of energy, substrates or signal molecules, to aid in the metabolism of lipids, glucose and cholesterols. However, SCFA generation, diet and bacterial composition are delicately interlinked. For example, diets with high fiber, low fat and high protein intake, lead to greater amounts of SCFAs than diets with reduced fiber content, thereby lowering the pH in the intestine and inhibiting the growth of pH-sensitive microbiota, that affects the production of SCFAs. Given the complexity of microbial metabolic pathways and cross-feeding mechanisms involved in SCFA production, there is not a simple linear correlation between intestinal SCFA levels and diet or microbial composition. Likewise, administration of a single dietary component or bacterial strain would unlikely result in an appreciable change in the concentration of SCFAs. Altogether, the intestinal microbiota essentially serves as 'external metabolic organ' that continuously supplies the host with absorbable nutrients and efficient energy.

Intestinal Epithelial Barrier and Homeostasis

Maintenance of intestinal homeostasis requires structural integrity of the epithelium. The intestinal epithelium in the healthy individual represents a semi-permeable physical barrier, on the one hand shielding the host from invasions of pathogens, and on the other hand allowing selective passage of nutrients. This is achieved thanks to a complex organization of the intestinal epithelium, which establishes a tightly regulated barrier [27]. The intestinal epithelium is built of columnar epithelial cells that are connected by tight junctions (Tjs), a multi-protein complex, which tightens the paracellular cleft, but also specifically regulates its permeability. During inflammation the intestinal epithelium can be easily disrupted and several effects on TJs have been observed; it generates an increased paracellular transport of solutes and water and an elevated permeability to large molecules including luminal pathogens [28] that has been evidenced in the beginning of IBD. This primary permeability defect was associated with increased secretion of interferon-γ and tumor necrosis factor (TNF)-α as inflammation developed.

It is important to mention that intestinal epithelium must be considered much more than a simple physical barrier, but it also has innate immune cell functions to actively combat pathogens through antimicrobial peptides and a protective mucus layer. The secretion of mucus and antimicrobial proteins by secretory cells (e.g., goblet cells and Paneth cells), provides a shield against antigens in the intestinal lumen [29].

Influence of the Gut Microbiota on Intestinal Barrier Integrity

Over the past years, several studies documented changes in the commensal gut microflora of patients with IBD [30], including a reduced complexity of commensals or a shift towards a specific phylum. It is still currently unclear whether these disturbances are cause or consequence of the manifestation of IBD. The intestinal microbiota represents the entirety of microorganisms in the human intestine and includes not only bacteria, but also fungi and viruses [31]. The most frequent microorganisms are commensal bacteria that are beneficial for the host, as they help to digest nutrients and compete with pathogens for the same ecological niches. To distinguish between harmful pathogens and beneficial commensals, intestinal epithelial cells and innate immune cells, such as dendritic cells and macrophages, are equipped with a variety of innate immune receptors, known as pathogen recognition receptors [32]. These findings support a disturbed microbiota in patients with IBD, which can be initiated because of a dysregulated epithelial-immune cell communication. The intestinal microbiota has demonstrated to be an important regulator of epithelial–immune cell communication and patients with IBD often show a dysbiosis. Shaping the gut microflora with specific probiotics is now seen as a supportive therapeutic approach in the treatment of IBD. Identifying important molecular interactions of the intestinal epithelium with the microbiota and the immune system influencing intestinal permeability and communication with the immune system will provide important insight into the pathogenesis of IBD and has potential to yield novel therapeutic approaches.

Dysbiosis and IBD

Any alteration in the balance or the composition of the microbiota is called dysbiosis. The composition of the microbiota depends on several factors including age, the dietary changes, genetic composition, response of the immune system of T and B cells, administration of antibiotics and chemotherapic drugs [13, 33].

The dramatic improvements to DNA sequencing technology and analysis over the last decade have set the stage for investigations of the IBD microbiome. Many studies find structural imbalances, or dysbioses, that occur in IBD since the initial report [34], and a broad pattern has begun to emerge, which includes a reduction in biodiversity, a decreased representation of several taxa within the *Firmicutes* phylum, and an increase in the *Gammaproteobacteria* [35].

Many studies consistently report a decrease in biodiversity, known as alpha-diversity or species richness in ecological terms, a measure of the total number of species in a community. There is a reduced alpha-diversity in the fecal microbiome in CD compared to healthy controls [36], which was also found in pairs of monozygotic twins discordant for CD [37].

This decreased diversity has been attributed to a reduced diversity specifically within the *Firmicutes* phylum [38], and has also been associated with temporal instability in the dominant taxa in both UC and CD [39]. There is a reduced diversity in inflamed versus non-inflamed tissues even within the same patient, and CD patients have lower overall bacterial loads at inflamed regions [40]. The largest IBD-related microbiome study to date, is on new-onset Crohn's disease in a multicenter pediatric cohort [41]. This study analyzed over 1000 treatment-nave samples, which were collected from multiple concurrent gastrointestinal locations, from patients representing the variety of disease phenotypes with respect to location, severity, and behavior. In addition to a detailed characterization of the specific organisms, either lost or associated with disease, this study indicates that assessing the rectal mucosa-associated microbiome offers unique potential for convenient and early diagnosis of CD.

Other non-bacterial members of the microbiota, namely the fungi, viruses, archaea, and phage may have a significant role in gastrointestinal disease [42]; however, the vast majority of recent studies of the microbiota are based on 16S sequencing, thus largely ignoring these groups of organisms. For example, norovirus infection, in the context of an intact gut microflora and mutated Atg16l1, is required for the development of CD in a mouse model [43].

Protective Effects of Microbes in IBD

Several lines of evidence suggest that specific groups of gut bacteria may have protective effects against IBD. For example, the colitis phenotype following treatment with dextran sulfate sodium is more severe in mice that are reared germ-free compared to conventionally reared mice [44]. One mechanism by which the commensal microbiota may protect the host is colonization resistance; commensals occupy niches within the host and prevent colonization by pathogens [45] and help out-compete pathogenic bacteria [46] (Interestingly, the microbiota can sometimes take on the opposite role and facilitate viral infection [47]).

Commensal microbiota can also have direct functional effects on potential pathogens, for example in dampening virulence-related gene expression [48]. In addition, the gut microbiota plays a role in shaping the mucosal immune system. *Bacteroides* and *Clostridium* species have been shown to induce the expansion of Treg cells, reducing intestinal inflammation [49]. Other members of the microbiota can attenuate mucosal inflammation by regulating nuclear factor (NF)-κ B activation [50].

Several bacterial species, most notably the *Bifidobacterium*, *Lactobacillus*, and *Faecalibacterium* genera, may protect the host from mucosal inflammation by several mechanisms, including the downregulation of inflammatory cytokines [51] or stimulation of IL-10 [52], an anti-inflammatory cytokine. *Faecalibacterium prausnitzii*, one such proposed member of the microbiota with anti-inflammatory properties, is under-represented in IBD [53].

F. prausnitzii is depleted in CD biopsy samples concomitant with an increase in *E. coli* abundance [54], and low levels of mucosa-associated *F. prausnitzii* are associated with higher risk of recurrent CD following surgery [52]. Conversely, recovery of *F. prausnitzii* after relapse is associated with maintenance of clinical remission of UC [55].

Several constituents of the gut microbiota ferment dietary fiber, a prebiotic, to produce short-chain fatty acids (SCFAs), which include acetate, propionate, and butyrate. SCFAs are the primary energy source for colonic epithelial cells [56] and have recently been shown to induce the expansion of colonic Treg cells [49]. The *Ruminococcacea*e, particularly the butyrate-producing genus *Faecalibacterium* [57], is decreased in IBD, especially in iCD [54]. Other SCFA-producing bacteria including *Odoribacter* and the *Leuconostocaceae* are reduced in UC, and *Phascolarctobacterium* and *Roseburia* are reduced in CD [35]. Interestingly, the *Ruminococcaceae* consume hydrogen and produce acetate that can be utilized by *Roseburia* to produce butyrate, and it is therefore consistent that both groups together are reduced in IBD.

IBD Treatments Affecting the Microbiome

In addition to environmental and dietary effects on the gut microbiome and their impact on IBD, some of the medications used in the treatment of IBD have inadvertent effects on the microbiome. An array of antibiotics has been shown to lead to a bloom of *Escherichia coli* [58]. Since increased *Enterobacteriaceae* is a distinctive feature of intestinal inflammation and oxidative stress, the relationship between microbial composition, inflammation, and antibiotic use forms an important topic for future research. In contrast, a meta-analysis of antibiotic use in IBD found that overall antibiotics had a beneficial effect [59]. However, it has been suggested that antibiotics may also play a direct role in the development of IBD by leading to dysbiosis and reduced bacterial diversity, this topic will require further controlled trials [60]. Will be required studies that monitor the temporal response at the levels of microbial ecology and functional composition [61] to understand the role of the microbiota in treatment outcome and the consequences of perturbing the gut microbiota of patients. Thus, several studies conducted in healthy humans, briefly exposed to some antibiotics, demonstrate the directly negative effect on the gastrointestinal epithelium and the spread of antibiotic resistant organisms [62]. Repeated exposures to a single antibiotic in healthy individuals results in cumulative and persistent changes to gut microbial composition [63].

Microbial homeostasis is typically disrupted by the loss of species complexity, particularly of protective microbes, thereby potentially resulting in an increased risk of infections [64], or dysbiosis [41]. Another mechanism, by which antibiotics lead to increased gut infections, is by causing a thinning of the mucus layer, thereby weakening its barrier function [65].

Fecal Microbiota Transplantation (FMT) in IBD

The discovery of the microbiome as a key component of both activation of innate immunity and maintenance of chronic inflammation in IBD has revealed an exciting and huge potential for an alternative and synergistic approach to current treatments.

Instead of perturbing the existing microbiome by removing diversity through antibiotics, repopulating the gut habitat with a healthy community has gained popularity in the last few years. This will be an exciting new direction for the pharmaceutical industry, expanding the focus beyond traditional small biologics [66]. The complexity and composition that will be used to repopulate the gut community will be very important. The success of probiotics in the management of IBD ranges from mixed results to considerable potential [67], and is dependent on the strains used and disease subtype targeted. It is important to mention, that none of the present generation of probiotics has been beneficial in CD; results have been more encouraging in UC, particularly patients with pouchitis and these are supplements, not substitutes or alternatives, for conventional therapy.

The efficacy of fecal microbiota transplantation (FMT) in patients with recurrent *Clostridium difficile* infection (CDI) has generated optimism for its use in IBD [68]. Initial data supporting a role for FMT in treating IBD came from small series, often in patients with a refractory disease. Related studies have shown that the use of a well-selected community subset, rather than whole fecal communities, can be sufficient for recovery [69]. The high success rate reported for relapsing CDI has elevated FMT as an emerging treatment for several gastrointestinal and metabolic disorders [70], and is actively being considered for IBD [71].

In conclusion, FMT is a safe and effective option in the short term to prevent recurrent CDI's in patients with IBD, and will likely remain an important tool in the future. The potential for microbial therapies to treat IBD seems promising; however, clinical development of reproducible microbial intervention to Food and Drug Administration (FDA) standards is currently lacking.

REFERENCES

[1] Loftus EV. (2004) Clinical epidemiology of inflammatory bowel disease: Incidence, prevalence, and environmental influences. *Gastroenterology. 126*:1504-1517.

[2] Oliva-Hemker M, Fiocchi C. (2002) Etiopathogenesis of inflammatory bowel disease: the importance of the pediatric perspective. *Inflamm Bowel Dis. 8*:112-128.

[3] Fiocchi C. (2002) Inflammatory bowel disease: dogmas and heresies. *Dig Liver Dis. 34*:306-311.

[4] Meucci G, Bortoli A, Riccioli FA, et al. (1999) Frequency and clinical evolution of indeterminate colitis: a retrospective multi-centre study in northern Italy. GSMII (Gruppo di Studio per le Malattie Infiammatorie Intestinali). *Eur J Gastroenterol Hepatol. 11:*909-13.

[5] Laroux FS, Pavlick KP, Wolf RE, et al. (2001) Dysregulation of intestinal mucosal immunity: implications in inflammatory bowel disease. *News Physiol Sci. 16*:272-277.
[6] Sands BE, Grabert S. (2009) Epidemiology of inflammatory bowel disease and overview of pathogenesis. *Med Health R I. 92*:73-77.
[7] Russell RK, Satsangi J. (2004) IBD: a family affair. *Best Pract Res Clin Gastroenterol. 18:*525-539.
[8] Baumgart DC, Carding SR. (2007) Inflammatory bowel disease: cause and immunobiology. *Lancet. 369*:1627-1640.
[9] Pillai S. (2013) Rethinking mechanisms of autoimmune pathogenesis. *J Autoimmun. 45*:97-103.
[10] Martín-de-Carpi J, Rodríguez A, Ramos E, et al. (2013) Increasing incidence of pediatric inflammatory bowel disease in Spain (1996-2009): the SPIRIT Registry. *Inflamm Bowel Dis. 19*:73-80.
[11] Spor A, Koren O, Ley R. (2011) Unravelling the effects of the environment and host genotype on the gut microbiome. *Nat Rev Microbiol. 9*:279-290.
[12] Dominguez-Bello MG, Blaser MJ, Ley RE, et al. (2011) Development of the human gastrointestinal microbiota and insights from high-throughput sequencing. *Gastroenterology. 140*:1713-1719.
[13] Lozupone CA, Stombaugh JI, Gordon JI, et al. (2012). Diversity, stability and resilience of the human gut microbiota. *Nature. 489*:220-230.
[14] Claesson MJ, Cusack S, O'Sullivan O, et al. (2011) Composition, variability, and temporal stability of the intestinal microbiota of the elderly. *Proc Natl Acad Sci U S A. 108*:4586-4591.
[15] Ley RE, Hamady M, Lozupone C, et al. (2008) Evolution of mammals and their gut microbes. *Science. 320*:1647-1651.
[16] Wu GD, Chen J, Hoffmann C, Bittinger K, et al. (2011) Linking long-term dietary patterns with gut microbial enterotypes. *Science. 334*:105-108.
[17] Zimmer J, Lange B, Frick JS, Sauer H, et al. (2012) A vegan or vegetarian diet substantially alters the human colonic faecal microbiota. *Eur J Clin Nutr. 66*:53-60.

[18] Moschen AR, Wieser V, Tilg H. (2012) Dietary Factors: Major Regulators of the Gut's Microbiota. *Gut Liver. 6*:411-416.
[19] Flint HJ, Scott KP, Louis P, et al. (2012) The role of the gut microbiota in nutrition and health. *Nat Rev Gastroenterol Hepatol. 9*:577-589.
[20] Baquero F, Nombela C. (2012) The microbiome as a human organ. *Clin Microbiol Infect. 18*:2-4.
[21] Dave M, Higgins PD, Middha S, et al. (2012) The human gut microbiome: current knowledge, challenges, and future directions. *Transl Res. 160*:246-257.
[22] Flint HJ, Scott KP, Duncan SH, et al. (2012) Microbial degradation of complex carbohydrates in the gut. *Gut Microbes. 3*:289-306.
[23] Krajmalnik-Brown R, Ilhan ZE, Kang DW, et al. (2012) Effects of gut microbes on nutrient absorption and energy regulation. *Nutr Clin Pract. 27*:201-214.
[24] Bergman EN. (1999) Energy contributions of volatile fatty acids from the gastrointestinal tract in various species. *Physiol Rev. 70*:567-590.
[25] Sonnenburg JL, Xu J, Leip DD, et al. (2005) Glycan foraging in vivo by an intestine-adapted bacterial symbiont. *Science. 307*:1955-1959.
[26] den Besten G, van Eunen K, Groen AK, et al. (2013) The role of short-chain fatty acids in the interplay between diet, gut microbiota, and host energy metabolism. *J Lipid Res. 54*:2325-2340.
[27] Mandel LJ, Bacallao R, Zampighi G. (1993) Uncoupling of the molecular 'fence' and paracellular 'gate' functions in epithelial tight junctions. *Nature. 361*:552-555.
[28] Fava F, Danese S. (2011) Intestinal microbiota in inflammatory bowel disease: friend of foe? *World J Gastroenterol. 17*:557-566.
[29] Donaldson GP, Lee SM, Mazmanian SK. (2016) Gut biogeography of the bacterial microbiota. *Nat Rev Microbiol. 14*:20-32.
[30] Matsuoka K, Kanai T. (2015) The gut microbiota and inflammatory bowel disease. *Semin Immunopathol. 37*:47-55.
[31] Plottel CS, Blaser MJ. (2011) Microbiome and malignancy. *Cell Host Microbe. 10*:324-335.
[32] Kelly D, Conway S, Aminov R. (2005) Commensal gut bacteria: mechanisms of immune modulation. *Trends Immunol. 26*:326-333.

[33] Parekh PJ, Balart LA, Johnson DA. (2015) The Influence of the Gut Microbiome on Obesity, Metabolic Syndrome and Gastrointestinal Disease. *Clin Transl Gastroenterol. 6*:e91.

[34] Frank DN, St Amand AL, Feldman RA, et al. (2007) Molecular-phylogenetic characterization of microbial community imbalances in human inflammatory bowel diseases. *Proc Natl Acad Sci USA. 104*:13780-13785.

[35] Morgan XC, Tickle TL, Sokol H, et al. (2012) Dysfunction of the intestinal microbiome in inflammatory bowel disease and treatment. *Genome Biol. 13*:R79.

[36] Manichanh C, Rigottier-Gois L, Bonnaud E, et al. (2006) Reduced diversity of faecal microbiota in Crohn's disease revealed by a metagenomic approach. *Gut. 55*:205-211.

[37] Dicksved J, Halfvarson J, Rosenquist M, et al. (2008) Molecular analysis of the gut microbiota of identical twins with Crohn's disease. *ISME J. 2*:716-727.

[38] Kang S, Denman SE, Morrison M, et al. (2010) Dysbiosis of fecal microbiota in Crohn's disease patients as revealed by a custom phylogenetic microarray. *Inflamm Bowel Dis. 16*:2034-2042.

[39] Martinez C, Antolin M, Santos J, et al. (2008) Unstable composition of the fecal microbiota in ulcerative colitis during clinical remission. *Am J Gastroenterol. 103*:643-648.

[40] Sepehri S, Kotlowski R, Bernstein CN, et al. (2007) Microbial diversity of inflamed and noninflamed gut biopsy tissues in inflammatory bowel disease. *Inflamm Bowel Dis. 13*:675-683.

[41] Gevers D, Kugathasan S, Denson LA, et al. (2014) The treatment-naive microbiome in new-onset Crohn's disease. *Cell Host Microbe. 15*:382-392.

[42] Hunter P. (2013) The secret garden's gardeners. Research increasingly appreciates the crucial role of gut viruses for human health and disease. *EMBO Rep. 14*:683-685.

[43] Cadwell K, Patel KK, Maloney NS, et al. (2010) Virus-plus-susceptibility gene interaction determines Crohn's disease gene Atg16L1 phenotypes in intestine. *Cell. 141*:1135-1145.

[44] Kitajima S, Morimoto M, Sagara E, et al. (2001) Dextran sodium sulfate-induced colitis in germ-free IQI/Jic mice. *Exp Anim. 50*:387-395.
[45] Callaway TR, Edrington TS, Anderson RC, et al. (2008) Probiotics, prebiotics and competitive exclusion for prophylaxis against bacterial disease. *Anim Health Res Rev. 9*:217-225.
[46] Kamada N, Chen G, Núñez G. (2012) A complex microworld in the gut: Harnessing pathogen-commensal relations. *Nat Med. 18*:1190-1191.
[47] Kane M, Case LK, Kopaskie K, et al. (2011) Successful transmission of a retrovirus depends on the commensal microbiota. *Science. 334*:245-249.
[48] Medellin-Peña MJ, Wang H, Johnson R, et al. (2007) Probiotics affect virulence-related gene expression in Escherichia coli O157:H7. *Appl Environ Microbiol. 73*:4259-4267.
[49] Atarashi K, Tanoue T, Oshima K, et al. (2013) Treg induction by a rationally selected mixture of Clostridia strains from the human microbiota. *Nature.500*:232-236.
[50] Kelly D, Campbell JI, King TP, et al. (2004) Commensal anaerobic gut bacteria attenuate inflammation by regulating nuclear-cytoplasmic shuttling of PPAR-gamma and RelA. *Nat Immunol. 5*:104-112.
[51] Llopis M, Antolin M, Carol M, et al. (2009) Lactobacillus casei downregulates commensals' inflammatory signals in Crohn's disease mucosa. *Inflamm Bowel Dis. 15*:275-283.
[52] Sokol H, Pigneur B, Watterlot L, et al. (2008) Faecalibacterium prausnitzii is an anti-inflammatory commensal bacterium identified by gut microbiota analysis of Crohn disease patients. *Proc Natl Acad Sci USA. 105*:16731-16736.
[53] Sokol H, Seksik P, Furet JP, et al. (2009) Low counts of Faecalibacterium prausnitzii in colitis microbiota. *Inflamm Bowel Dis. 15*:1183-1189.
[54] Willing B, Halfvarson J, Dicksved J, et al. (2009) Twin studies reveal specific imbalances in the mucosa-associated microbiota of patients with ileal Crohn's disease. *Inflamm Bowel Dis. 15*:653-660.

[55] Varela E, Manichanh C, Gallart M, et al. (2013) Colonisation by Faecalibacterium prausnitzii and maintenance of clinical remission in patients with ulcerative colitis. *Aliment Pharmacol Ther. 38*:151-161.

[56] Ahmad MS, Krishnan S, Ramakrishna BS, et al. (2000) Butyrate and glucose metabolism by colonocytes in experimental colitis in mice. *Gut. 46*:493-499.

[57] Duncan SH, Hold GL, Barcenilla A, et al. (2002) Roseburia intestinalis sp. nov., a novel saccharolytic, butyrate-producing bacterium from human faeces. *Int J Syst Evol Microbiol. 52*:1615-1620.

[58] Looft T, Allen HK. (2012) Collateral effects of antibiotics on mammalian gut microbiomes. *Gut Microbes. 3*:463-467.

[59] Modi SR, Lee HH, Spina CS, et al. (2013) Antibiotic treatment expands the resistance reservoir and ecological network of the phage metagenome. *Nature. 499*:219-222.

[60] Khan KJ, Ullman TA, Ford AC, et al. (2011) Antibiotic therapy in inflammatory bowel disease: a systematic review and meta-analysis. *Am J Gastroenterol. 106*:661-673.

[61] Lemon KP, Armitage GC, Relman DA, et al. (2012) Microbiota-targeted therapies: an ecological perspective. *Sci Transl Med. 4*:137rv5.

[62] Relman DA. (2012) The human microbiome: ecosystem resilience and health. *Nutr Rev. 70*:S2-S9.

[63] Dethlefsen L, Relman DA. (2011) Incomplete recovery and individualized responses of the human distal gut microbiota to repeated antibiotic perturbation. *Proc Natl Acad Sci USA. 108*:4554-4561.

[64] Khosravi A, Mazmanian SK. (2013) Disruption of the gut microbiome as a risk factor for microbial infections. *Curr Opin Microbiol. 16*:221-227.

[65] Wlodarska M, Willing B, Keeney KM, et al. (2011) Antibiotic treatment alters the colonic mucus layer and predisposes the host to exacerbated Citrobacter rodentium-induced colitis. *Infect Immun. 79*:1536-1545.

[66] Fischbach MA, Bluestone JA, Lim WA. (2013) Cell-based therapeutics: the next pillar of medicine. *Sci Transl Med.* 5:179ps7.
[67] Whelan K, Quigley EM. (2013) Probiotics in the management of irritable bowel syndrome and inflammatory bowel disease. *Curr Opin Gastroenterol.* 29:184-189.
[68] van Nood E, Vrieze A, Nieuwdorp M, et al. (2013) Duodenal infusion of donor feces for recurrent Clostridium difficile. *N Engl J Med.* 368:407-415.
[69] Shahinas D, Silverman M, Sittler T, et al. (2012) Toward an understanding of changes in diversity associated with fecal microbiome transplantation based on 16S rRNA gene deep sequencing. *MBio. 3.*
[70] Smits LP, Bouter KE, de Vos WM, et al. (2013) Therapeutic potential of fecal microbiota transplantation. *Gastroenterology.* 145:946-953.
[71] Damman CJ, Miller SI, Surawicz CM, et al. (2012) The microbiome and inflammatory bowel disease: is there a therapeutic role for fecal microbiota transplantation? *Am J Gastroenterol.* 107:1452-1459.

In: Advances in Health and Disease
Editor: Lowell T. Duncan
ISBN: 978-1-53613-020-1
© 2018 Nova Science Publishers, Inc.

Chapter 8

SUDDEN DEATH

Luca Roncati[*]*, Antonio Manenti* *and Giuseppe Barbolini*

From the Departments of Pathology and Surgery, University of Modena and Reggio Emilia, Modena (MO), Italy

ABSTRACT

Sudden death can be defined as an unexpected event that happens in healthy people or in stable patients. It must occur within one hour from the onset of the first symptoms, and it is precipitated by a cardiac arrest, which is irreversible for the absence of an adequate and prompt assistance or for an intrinsic cardiac disease.

Heart block is usually preceded by severe disturbances of the cardiac rhythm, as ventricular fibrillation or bradycardia. In a first group of diseases, at the basis of this event, a primitive disorder, directly correlated with an abnormality of cell membrane channels involved in the exchange of electrolytes, can be found, as in Brugada's syndrome.

A more common condition is represented by infarct or severe ischemia, sometimes known before, that determine significant alterations in the cardiac rhythm, followed by ventricular fibrillation and cardiac arrest.

---

[*] Corresponding Author E-mail: emailmedical@gmail.com.

Rarer is an acute hemopericardium, where a sudden severe haemorrhage takes place inside the pericardium, with a primary effect of acute cardiac tamponade; in absence of recent cardio-thoracic surgery, a cause can be the rupture of an aortic aneurysm, involving its first intrapericardic tract.

Many other cardiac diseases, as acute myocarditis, left ventricular hypertrophy, hypertrophic cardiomyopathy, dilatative cardiomyopathy, restrictive cardiomyopathy, Arrhythmogenic Right Ventricular Cardiomyopathy (ARVC), pulmonary or aortic stenosis, atrial myxoma, and, rarely, Cyanotic Congenital Heart Diseases (CCHD), can induce a sudden cardiac arrest.

In other conditions, the cardiac arrest follows an acute primary disease of one or multiple apparatuses. At first, an abrupt and massive haemorrhage, followed by a fall in the venous return, can produce an electro-mechanical cardiac dissociation, with subsequent cardiac arrest. A similar condition is represented by anaphylactic shock, where a sudden peripheral vasodilatation with an abrupt fall in blood venous return can be associated with an increased pulmonary vascular resistance, bronchospasm and coronary vasoconstriction by circulating histamine. A characteristic condition is the onset of an acute respiratory failure, followed by acute hypoxia, hypercapnia and acidosis. It can happen after tension pneumothorax, complicating a respiratory insufficiency, or in case of bilateral pneumothorax.

Moreover, a sudden increase in pulmonary resistance accompanied by severe hypoxia, as in acute thrombo-embolism of the pulmonary artery, can determine a sudden cardiac arrest. Another cause, even rarer, of cardiac arrest is finally represented by a spontaneous cerebral haemorrhage, where a rapid rise of intracranial pressure, but more often a direct damage of vital cerebral centres, leads to a direct acute cardio-respiratory failure.

Keywords: sudden death, Brugada's syndrome, Wolff-Parkinson-White syndrome, Waterhouse-Friderichsen syndrome, Arrhythmogenic Right Ventricular Cardiomyopathy, anaphylactic shock

INTRODUCTION

Sudden death is considered a fatal not traumatic event that occurs in the short time of one hour after the unexpected arise of an acute disease (or its complications) in clinically stable patients; the death can follow directly or after an unsuccessful urgent treatment. The most common cause of sudden death is represented by a fatal cardiac arrest, correlated to an underlying disorder.

Cardiac arrest can be the expression of an irreversible change in the cardiac rhythm, which leads to ventricular fibrillation. A typical example of this is the Brugada's syndrome, an intrinsic disease, often congenital, of the conduction system. Here, a basal dysfunction of channels deputy to ions transport (mainly sodium and potassium), across the external cell membrane, is considered the trigger factor [1-3]. A similar condition is represented by the long or short QT syndromes, congenital or secondary to pharmacological treatments, and the Catecholaminergic Polymorphic Ventricular Tachycardia (CPVT). All these induce an increased cardiac excitability, with different clinical expression, like "torsade de pointes", which is a classic example of life-threating arrhythmia, often secondary to assumption of various drugs or related to disorders of plasma electrolytes [4, 5]. The above-mentioned conditions show typical electrocardiographic features, but not correspondent histopathological findings on autopsy, hence the term *white death*. "Torsade de pointes" can also occur in patient affected by Wolff-Parkinson-White syndrome, which is characterized by the congenital presence of the Kent's bundle, an abnormal extra or accessory conduction pathway between atria and ventricles [6].

Similarly, a healthy cardiac conduction system can be infiltrated by pathological tissue, as in course of lymphoma or sarcoidosis (Figure 1), so deeply impairing its normal function. Another group of dangerous diseases is represented by those involving the myocardium, in which its functional capacity is quickly and severely deteriorated, until an acute cardiac failure. It mainly regards the different forms of cardiomyopathies, that is hypertrophic, dilatative, restrictive or arrhythmogenic (Figure 2), and acute myocarditis (Figure 3). In these cases, a sudden death can follow an acute decrease of the left ventricle ejection fraction or a superimposed arrhythmia. An autoptic examine, with accurate histology, can allow an exact diagnosis.

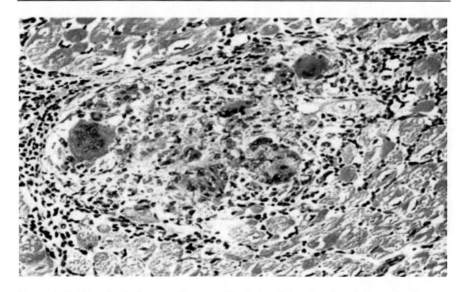

Figure 1. Sudden death from cardiac sarcoidosis involving the electrical conduction system of the heart: the non-necrotizing granulomatous inflammation is noticeable (Haematoxylin Eosin stain).

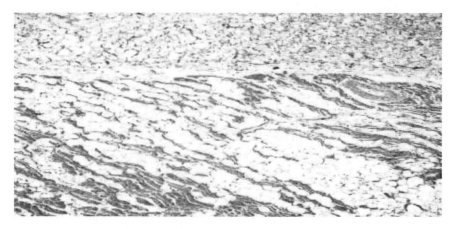

Figure 2. Sudden death from Arrhythmogenic Right Ventricular Cardiomyopathy (ARVC): a diffuse fatty infiltration of the right cardiac ventricle is visible (Hematoxylin Eosin stain).

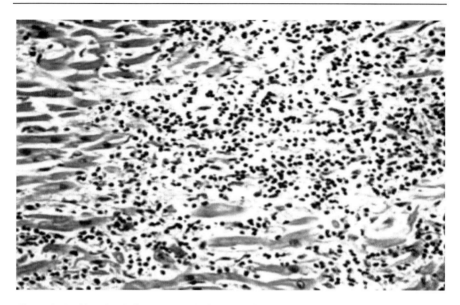

Figure 3. Sudden death from acute viral myocarditis: the dense lymphocytic infiltrate disrupts the cardiac muscle fibers (Hematoxylin Eosin stain).

Certainly, the most common cause of sudden cardiac death is an acute coronary insufficiency, due to atherosclerotic thrombosis and embolism or to non-atherosclerotic spasms. It acts promoting an acute alteration of the cardiac rhythm, as sinus node arrest or complete heart block, or favouring the final appearance of ventricular fibrillation. Sometimes, an acute cardiac dysfunction can quickly follow, especially when one or both ventricles are largely damaged. In all these cases, a sudden death often occurs, especially if an adequate treatment has not been implemented or the resuscitation manoeuvres have not been successful [7-9]. Congenital anomalies of the coronary arteries' origin or of the cardiac valves, such as Ebstein's anomaly, are considered predisposing factors [10]. In some cases of sudden death, after an acute myocardial infarct, the macroscopic findings at autopsy are scant, and the microscopical examination highlights a simple vacuolization of the sub-endocardial cells [11].

A further condition of sudden death is represented by cardiac tamponade, secondary to a haemorrhagic pericarditis or to an acute hemopericardium from intra-pericardial rupture of an aortic dissection

(Figure 4) or aortic aneurysm [12, 13]. The possible diseases at the basis of these complications could have been passed without an adequate diagnosis.

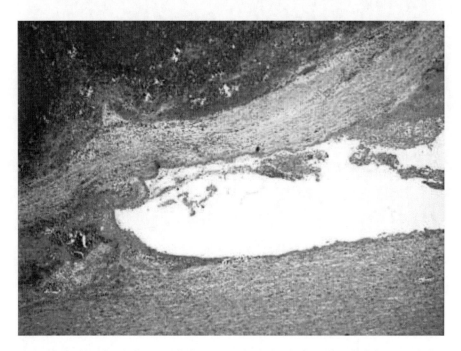

Figure 4. Sudden death from cardiac tamponade due to intra-pericardial rupture of an aortic dissection: note the conspicuous accumulation of extravasated blood (Hematoxylin Eosin stain).

Another condition leading to a sudden death can be an acute pulmonary hypertension, with the mechanism of an acute hypertension in the right ventricle. This typically happens during acute pulmonary venous thromboembolism or tension pneumothorax [14]. The diagnosis, especially in the first case, although clinically suspected, demand an autoptic control.

A particular cause of sudden cardiac arrest is represented by an acute and drastic decrease of the venous return to the heart. It can be secondary to conspicuous haemorrhage (e.g., digestive haemorrhage, massive pulmonary bleeding, extra-uterine pregnancy rupture), whose typical signs, however, appear usually before the onset of an electro-mechanical dissociation of the cardiac function [15]. A similar condition is represented by anaphylactic shock (Figure 5), with a sudden and complete vasodilation in the whole capillary system, and an abrupt fall of the blood pressure and venous return. The bronchospasm, often associated (Figure 6), with a subsequent respiratory insufficiency and an increase in pulmonary resistance, can precipitate the cardiac arrest, through a mechanism of hypercapnia-acidosis [16].

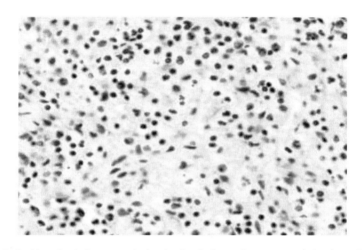

Figure 5. Sudden death from anaphylactic shock due to intravenous injection of antibiotics: many splenic degranulated mastocytes are well observable (Pagoda Red stain).

Excluding the possible causes of sudden death in foetuses and infants [17-26], we have to remember two causes of sudden death in adults, not directly correlated to a cardiac accident, but to neurological events. It regards the rupture of a subarachnoid aneurysm, which can precipitate the patient in a comatose state. When an adequate vital support is not supplied, a cardiac arrest follows in a short period of time. The same fatal evolution can follow an acute ischemic attack, especially if involving a large brain zone, brainstem or cerebellum. In particular, cerebellar infarct leads to a brainstem compression for marked swelling and oedema, with an increased intracranial pressure [27]. Many other diseases differently responsible of coma, such as fulminant hepatitis or meningitis, Waterhouse-Friderichsen syndrome (Figure 7), necrotizing acute pancreatitis [28], can cause the patient's death, which can be considered sudden, when the underlying disease is not recognized and the patient not promptly assisted.

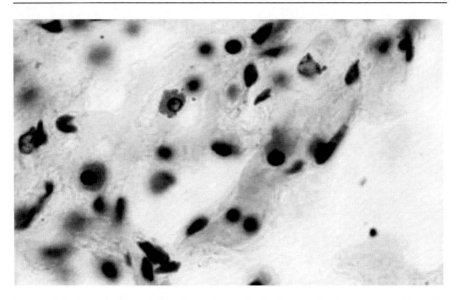

Figure 6. Sudden death from anaphylactic shock: the degranulated mastocytes (detail) are at the basis of the spasm, which involves the respiratory tract (Pagoda Red stain).

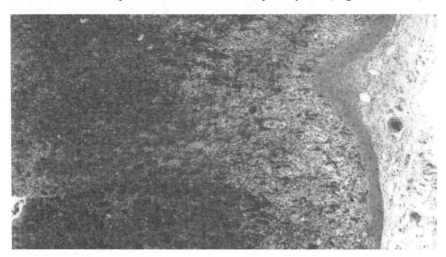

Figure 7. Sudden death from Waterhouse-Friderichsen syndrome: the adrenal hemorrhage has been triggered by pneumococcal sepsis (Hematoxylin Eosin stain).

REFERENCES

[1] Curcio, A., Santarpia, G., Indolfi, C. The Brugada syndrome - from gene to therapy. *Circ. J.* 2017; 81(3):290-7.

[2] Bastiaenen, R., Behr, E. R. Sudden death and ion channel disease: pathophysiology and implications for management. *Heart.* 2011; 97(17):1365-72.

[3] Goldenberg, I., Moss, A. J., Zareba, W. Sudden cardiac death without structural heart disease: update on the long QT and Brugada syndromes. *Curr. Cardiol. Rep.* 2005; 7(5):349-56.

[4] Roden, D. M. Clinical practice. Long-QT syndrome. *N. Engl. J. Med.* 2008; 358(2):169-76.

[5] Schimpf, R., Veltmann, C., Wolpert, C., Borggrefe, M. Arrhythmogenic hereditary syndromes: Brugada Syndrome, long QT syndrome, short QT syndrome and CPVT. *Minerva Cardioangiol.* 2010; 58(6):623-36.

[6] Kobza, R., Kottkamp, H., Hindricks, G. Images in cardiovascular medicine. Torsade de pointes in a patient with Wolff-Parkinson-White syndrome. *Circulation.* 2005; 111(13):e173-4.

[7] Aro, A. L., Rusinaru, C., Uy-Evanado, A., Reinier, K., Phan, D., Gunson, K., Jui, J., Chugh, S. S. Syncope and risk of sudden cardiac arrest in coronary artery disease. *Int. J. Cardiol.* 2017; 231:26-30.

[8] Glinge, C., Sattler, S., Jabbari, R., Tfelt-Hansen, J. Epidemiology and genetics of ventricular fibrillation during acute myocardial infarction. *J. Geriatr. Cardiol.* 2016; 13(9):789-97.

[9] Efferth, T., Banerjee, M., Paul, N. W. Broken heart, tako-tsubo or stress cardiomyopathy? Metaphors, meanings and their medical impact. *Int. J. Cardiol.* 2017; 230:262-8.

[10] Cheitlin, M. D., MacGregor, J. Congenital anomalies of coronary arteries: role in the pathogenesis of sudden cardiac death. *Herz.* 2009; 34(4):268-79.

[11] Mondello, C., Cardia, L., Ventura-Spagnolo, E. Immunohistochemical detection of early myocardial infarction: a systematic review. *Int. J. Legal. Med.* 2017; 131(2):411-21.

[12] Papagiannis, J. Sudden death due to aortic pathology. *Cardiol. Young.* 2017; 27(S1):S36-S42.
[13] Manenti, A., Roncati, L. A new look inside the pathogenesis of the thoracic aortic aneurysm. *Ann. Thorac. Surg.* 2013; 96(3):1124-5.
[14] Roncati, L., Pusiol, T., Piscioli, F., Scialpi, M., Barbolini, G., Maiorana, A. Pneumothorax-associated fibroblastic lesion in combination with localized pleural angiomatosis: a possible cause of juvenile spontaneous hemopneumothorax. *Pathol. Res. Pract.* 2015; 211(6):481-4.
[15] Zizzo, M., Roncati, L., Colasanto, D., Manenti, A. Pancolorectal varices superimposed on arteriovenous malformations: a life-threating complex disease. *Clin. Res. Hepatol. Gastroenterol.* 2016; 40(6):e75-6.
[16] Roncati, L., Barbolini, G., Scacchetti, A. T., Busani, S., Maiorana, A. Unexpected death: anaphylactic intraoperative death due to Thymoglobulin carbohydrate excipient. *Forensic. Sci. Int.* 2013; 228(1-3):e28-32.
[17] Roncati, L., Pusiol, T., Piscioli, F., Barbolini, G., Maiorana, A., Lavezzi, A. The first 5-year-long survey on intrauterine unexplained sudden deaths from the Northeast Italy. *Fetal. Pediatr. Pathol.* 2016; 35(5):315-26.
[18] Pusiol, T., Roncati, L., Lavezzi, A. M., Taddei, F., Piscioli, F., Ottaviani, G. Sudden fetal death due to dualism of the sino-atrial node. *Cardiovasc. Pathol.* 2016; 25(4):325-8.
[19] Roncati, L., Pusiol, T., Piscioli, F., Lavezzi, A. M. Neurodevelopmental disorders and pesticide exposure: the northeastern Italian experience. *Arch. Toxicol.* 2017; 91(2):603-4.
[20] Roncati, L, Termopoli, V., Pusiol, T. Negative role of the environmental endocrine disruptors in the human neurodevelopment. *Front. Neurol.* 2016; 7:143.
[21] Roncati, L., Piscioli, F., Pusiol, T. The endocrine disruptors among the environmental risk factors for stillbirth. *Sci. Total Environ.* 2016; 563-564:1086-7.

[22] Roncati, L., Piscioli, F., Pusiol, T. The endocrine disrupting chemicals as possible stillbirth contributors. *Am. J. Obstet. Gynecol.* 2016; 215(4):532-3.

[23] Lavezzi, A. M., Ferrero, S., Matturri, L., Roncati, L., Pusiol, T. Developmental neuropathology of brainstem respiratory centers in unexplained stillbirth: what's the meaning? *Int. J. Dev. Neurosci.* 2016; 53:99-106.

[24] Lavezzi, A. M., Ferrero, S., Roncati, L., Matturri, L., Pusiol, T. Impaired orexin receptor expression in the Kölliker-Fuse nucleus in sudden infant death syndrome: possible involvement of this nucleus in arousal pathophysiology. *Neurol. Res.* 2016; 38(8):706-16.

[25] Roncati, L., Barbolini, G., Pusiol, T., Piscioli, F., Maiorana, A. New advances on placental hydrops and related villous lymphatics. *Lymphology.* 2015; 48(1):28-37.

[26] Roncati, L., Barbolini, G., Fano, R. A., Rivasi, F. Fatal Aspergillus flavus infection in a neonate. *Fetal. Pediatr. Pathol.* 2010; 29(4):239-44.

[27] Stevens, R. D., Bhardwaj, A. Approach to the comatose patient. *Crit. Care Med.* 2006; 34(1):31-41.

[28] Roncati, L., Gualandri, G., Fortuni, G., Barbolini, G. Sudden death and lipomatous infiltration of the heart involved by fat necrosis resulting from acute pancreatitis. *Forensic Sci. Int.* 2012; 217(1-3):e19-22.

In: Advances in Health and Disease
Editor: Lowell T. Duncan

ISBN: 978-1-53613-020-1
© 2018 Nova Science Publishers, Inc.

Chapter 9

AMANTADINE FOR PARKINSON'S DISEASE

Shaheen E. Lakhan, MD, PhD, MEd, and Muhammad Safwatullah, MBBS*

ABSTRACT

From a single case use in 1969, amantadine has been shown to be efficacious in the treatment of Parkinson's disease and its complications. As a tricyclic amine, it enhances the release of dopamine at the synaptic cleft and inhibits its uptake, acts directly at the D2 receptor and up-regulates it, has anti-muscarinic properties, and non-competitive antagonism of the NMDA receptor. It has been studied as both a monotherapy or adjuvant therapy for Parkinson's disease with mixed results. Likewise, it has been investigated for other neurodegenerative conditions such as multiple system atrophy, progressive supranuclear palsy, and other akinetic-rigid syndromes. Its long-term effects are being delineated.

---

* Corresponding Author E-mail: slakhan@gnif.org

INTRODUCTION

Amantadine, originally approved as an antiviral agent, has gained its significance in the scientific community as a treatment for Parkinson's disease. It was incidentally discovered to improve the rigidity, tremor, and akinesia of Parkinson's disease in a 58-year-old woman taking amantadine to prevent influenza (Schwab et al., 1969). Since that time, a considerable number of studies have been performed to corroborate the role of amantadine in Parkinson's disease.

MECHANISM OF ACTION

The mechanism of action of amantadine in Parkinson's disease has been studied since early 1970's. Early in vitro research suggests that amantadine acts on central dopamine and noradrenaline neurons presynaptically. It releases DA and NA from extragranular sites close to the nerve terminal (Farnebo et al., 1971) and it antagonizes DA uptake (Heikila and Cohen, 1972). In addition, it also has mild anticholinergic effects (Nastuk et al., 1976). However, later studies have revealed that amantadine is a non-competitive NMDA receptor antagonist (Korhuber et al., 1991). The excitotoxic effects of NMDA receptors enhance degeneration of dopaminergic neurons in the substantia nigra. It has been speculated that the antiparkinsonian (Kornhuber et al., 1991), neuroprotective (Uitti et al, 1996), and antidyskinetic (Chase et al., 1996; Calon et al., 2002) properties of amantadine are mainly due to NMDA receptor antagonism. Antagonizing these receptors in the basal ganglia may have a pivotal role in providing "levodopa-sparing" therapeutic options to patients with Parkinson's disease.

AMANTADINE IN THE TREATMENT OF PARKINSON'S DISEASE

Although amantadine undoubtedly improved symptoms of Parkinson's, it took a back seat in the treatment of Parkinson's disease for many years. This is mainly because it was thought to have only a "transient benefit," which meant that the effect of the drug lasted only for 6-12 months due to a rapid decrease in response following administration known as tachyphylaxis (Factor and Molho, 1999). This generalization might have emerged from one of the initial studies on amantadine conducted by Schwab et al. In this study, marked improvement was noted in patients taking amantadine for three to eight months and some of these patients showed a reduced improvement after the first 4-8 weeks. Another study using an ergometer to measure akinesia reported the peak effect of amantadine in the first week with a return of the ergometer score to baseline after three months (Timberlake and Vance, 1978).

Additional studies have shown different results. The twenty-six patients selected to receive amantadine only in a study by Parkes et al., (1970) saw sustained improvement for a one-year period. A study by Zeldowicz et al, (1973) selected seventy-seven patients at different stages of Parkinson's disease for long-term amantadine treatment. Nineteen of these patients showed continued improvement for over twenty-one months. The difference in these results may be due to individual variability and progression of disease.

Other aspects of amantadine treatment have also been considered. A greater proportion of controlled trials have been designed to observe the use of amantadine alone or with other antiparkinsonian drugs. According to Forssman et al., (1972), amantadine has shown improvement in all facets of Parkinson's disease when given alone or when added to anticholinergics. When comparing benzhexol and amantadine, Parkes et al. (1974) noted that benzhexol treatment gave a slight improvement in rigidity and flexion deformity whereas amantadine had a very slight effect on akinesia and a moderate improvement in both tremor and posture. Moreover, combined benzhexol and amantadine treatment improved all symptoms. Hence, depending on the disability and response of the individual, amantadine may be of clinical use alone or as an adjunct with anticholinergics prior to levodopa treatment.

Most common approach in studying amantadine treatment has been to compare its effects with levodopa, the most efficacious treatment for Parkinson's disease (Rezak, 2007). Zeldowicz et al., (973) has reported an improvement in the functional level as well as symptoms in nineteen out of seventy-seven patients taking amantadine without levodopa. The neurological deficits (tremor, rigidity, akinesia, speech and salivation) were not as severe in these patients as those chosen for levodopa and amantadine therapy. Amantadine produced further improvement in the thirty-seven patients taking both levodopa and amantadine. Parkes et al., (1971) chose to add on levodopa after three months of amantadine to patients who needed additional treatment and did not have adequate control of their symptoms with amantadine alone. Most studies have concluded that amantadine alone is sufficient in those with mild to moderate disability.

Another factor being questioned in recent amantadine research is in the treatment of levodopa induced dyskinesias (LID). Controlled trials have continually showed a reduction in dyskinesias (Verhagen et al., 1999; Luginger et al., 2000; Thomas et al., 2004; Wolf et al., 2010). A reduction in severity and duration of daily off-time has been observed by Verhagen et al., (1998). In this study, scores for dyskinesia were obtained after three weeks of amantadine treatment in patients given intravenous levodopa infusions. Another five-week study by Luginger et al., (2000) also confirmed reduced intensity in LID study in patients who were administered levodopa orally. These short-term trials have become the basis of longer studies.

Long-term trials of amantadine use in the treatment of LID have shown varying results. Verhagen et al., (1999) and Wolf et al., (2010) have demonstrated a sustained reduction of dyskinesia for one year or more. However, Thomas et al., reported peak effect of amantadine after 15 days and a loss of effect at three to eight months. This study was designed for the duration of one year, but ended early nine months because an improvement with amantadine was no longer detected. Therefore, the role of amantadine in the armamentarium against Parkinson's disease is still being defined.

AMANTADINE IN OTHER AKINETIC RIGID SYNDROMES

Amantadine's applicability in Parkinson's disease has extended its search for use in other Parkinson syndromes. In multiple system atrophy, it has not shown a clinically significant reduction of akinesia, rigidity, tremor, postural instability, and gait disorder (Wenning, 2005). Another Parkinson syndrome in which it has not shown a significant improvement is in progressive supranuclear palsy (Rajput et al., 1997). Although, some symptoms of these disorders overlap with those of idiopathic Parkinson's, these neurodegenerative disorders involve structures other than the basal ganglia. Therefore, the mechanism of amantadine in these syndromes is still unclear.

CONCLUSION

Although many aspects of amantadine treatment have yet to be defined, it is undeniable that it has some benefit in Parkinson's disease. Its mode of action as well as duration of improvement in parkinsonian and levodopa-induced dyskinetic symptoms continue to be studied to this day. After being studied extensively, it is usually prescribed to control symptoms early in the disease to delay treatment with levodopa. In later stages of the disease, it may also be added to levodopa to reduce dyskinesias. Amantadine is preferred due to its relatively low side effects. It has recently been approved in extended-release capsules for the treatment of Parkinson's disease, mostly in the setting of levodopa-induced dyskinesias.

REFERENCES

Calon, F.; Morissette, Marc; Ghirbi, O.; Goulet, M.; Grondin; R.; Blanchet, P. J.; Bedard, P. J.; Paolo, T. D. Alteration of glutamate receptors in the striatum of dyskinetic 1-methyl-4-phenyl-1, 2, 3,6-tetrahydropyridine-treated monkeys following dopamine agonist treatment. *Progress in Neuro-Psychopharmacology & Biological Psychiatry, 2002* 26, 127-138.

Chase, T. N.; Engber, T. M.; Mouradian M. M. Contribution of dopaminergic and glutaminergic mechanisms to the pathogenesis of motor response complications in Parkinson's disease. *Adv. Neurol.,* 1996 69, 497-501.

Factor, S. A.; Molho, E. S. Transient benefit of amantadine in Parkinson's disease: the facts about the myth. *Movement Disorders,* 1999 14, 515-517.

Farnebo, L. O.; Fuxe, K., Goldstein, M.; Hamberger, B.; Ungerstedt, U. Dopamine and noradrenaline releasing action of amantadine in the central and peripheral nervous system; a possible mode of action in Parkinson's disease. *European Journal of Pharmacology,* 1971 16, 27-38.

Forssman, B.; Kihlstrand, S.; Larsson, L. E. Amantadine therapy in Parkinsonism. *Acta Neurologica Scandinavica.* 1972 48, 1-18.

Gianutsos, G.; Chute, S.; Dunn, J. P. Pharmacological changes in dopaminergic systems induced by long-term administration of amantadine. *European Journal of Pharmacology,* 1985 110, 357-361.

Heikkila, R. E.; Cohen, G. Evaluation of amantadine as a releasing agent or uptake blocker ^{3}H-dopamine in rat brain slices. *European J. Pharmacology,* 1972 20, 156.

Kornhuber, J.; Bormann, J.; Retz, W.; Hubers, M.; Reiderer, P. Effects of the 1-amino-adamantanes at the MK-801-binding site of the NMDA-receptor-gated ion channel –a human postmortem brain study. *European Journal of Pharmacology,* 1989 206, 297-300.

Luginger, E.; Wenning, G. K.; Bosch, S.; Poewe, W. Beneficial effects of amantadine on L-dopa-induced dyskinesias in Parkinson's disease. *Movement Disorders*, 2000 15,873-878.

Nastuk, W. L.; Su, P. C.; Doubilet, P. Anticholinergic and membrane activities of amantadine in neuromuscular transmission. *Nature*, 1976 264, 76-79.

Parkes, J. D.; Curzon, G.; Knott, P. J.; Tattersall, R.; Baxter, R. C. H.; Knill-Jones, R. P.; Marsden, C. D.; Vollum, Dorothy. Treatment of Parkinson's disease with amantadine and levodopa: a one year study. *The Lancet*, 1971 I, 1083-1087.

Parkes, J. D.; Baxter, R. C.; Mardsen, C. D.; Rees, J. E. Comparative trial of benzhexol, amantadine, and levodopa in the treatment of Parkinson's disease. *Journal of Neurology, Neruosurgery, and Psychiatry*, 1974 37, 422-426.

Rajput, A. H.; Uitti, R. J.; Fenton, M. E.; Georges, D. Amantadine effectiveness in multiple system atrophy and progressive supranuclear palsy. *Parkinsonism & Related Disorders*, 1998 3, 211-214.

Rezak, M. Current pharmacotherapeutic treatment options in Parkinson's Disease. *Disease-A-Month Journal*, 2007 53, 214-222.

Schwab, RS; England AC; Poskanzer, DC; Young, RR. Amantadine in the treatment of Parkinson's disease. *Jama,* 1969 208, 1168-1170.

Thomas, A.; Lacano, D.; Luciano, A. L.; Armellino, K.; Di lorio, A.; Onofj, M. duration of amantadine benefit on dyskinesia of severe Parkinson's disease. *J. Neruol. Neurosurg. Psychiatry,* 2004 75, 141-143.

Timberlake, W. H.; Vance M. A. Four-year Treatment of patients with Parkinsonism using amantadine alone or with levodopa. *Annals of Neurology,* 1978 3, 119-128.

Verhagen Metman, L.; Del Dotto, P.; van den, M. P.; Fang, J.; Mouradian N. M.; Chase, TN. Amantadine as treatment for dyskinesia and motor fluctuations in Parkinson's disease. *Neurology*, 1998 50, 1323-1326.

Verhagen Metman, L.; Del Dott, P.; LePoole, K.; Konisiotis, S.; Fang, J.; Chase, T. N. Amantadine for levodopa-induced dyskinesias: a 1-year follow-up study. *Arch. Neurol.*, 1999 56, 1383-1386.

Wenning, G. K. Placebo-controlled trial of amantadine in multiple-system atrophy. *Clinical Neuropharmacology,* 2005 28, 225-227.

Wolf, E.; Seppi, K.; Katzenschlager, R.; Hochschorner, G.; Ransmayr, G.; Schwingenschuh, P.; Ott, E.; Kloiber, I.; Haubenberger, D.; Auff, E.; Poewe, W. Long-term antidyskinetic efficacy of amantadine in Parkinson's disease. *Movement Disorders,* 2010 25, 1357-1363.

Zeldowicz, L. R.; Huberman, J.; Vancouver, B. .C. Long-term therapy of Parkinson's disease with amantadine, alone and combined with levodopa. *CMA Journal,* 1973 109, 588-593.

INDEX

A

acetabulum, 150, 154, 155, 156, 157, 163, 165
acid, 11, 13, 16, 21, 84, 107, 116
acidosis, xv, 218, 223
acquired immunodeficiency syndrome, 188
acute myocarditis, xiv, 218, 219
adherence, vii, xi, 120, 124, 127, 128, 129, 130, 131, 132, 134, 135, 136, 137, 138, 139, 140, 141, 143, 145
adipokinetic hormone, ix, 2, 3, 4, 31, 34, 36, 38, 39, 42, 43
akinesia, 230, 231, 232, 233
Akinetic Rigid Syndromes, 233
alexithymia, 138
alkaline phosphatase, 23, 31, 178
alters, 200, 211, 215
amantadine, vi, 229, 230, 231, 232, 233, 234, 235
amino, 9, 11, 15, 16, 18, 25, 28, 33, 38, 42, 95, 98, 234
anaerobic bacteria, 202
anaphylactic shock, xv, 218, 222, 223, 224
anatomy, xi, xii, 149, 150, 151, 154, 165, 166

aneurysm, xiv, 218, 222, 223, 226
antagonism, viii, xv, 20, 229, 230
antibiotic, 208, 214
anticholinergic effect, 230
antidepressant, 117, 146
antihypertensive agents, 140
anxiety, 68, 124, 126, 129
aortic aneurysm, xiv, 218, 222, 226
aortic dissection, 221, 222
aortic stenosis, xiv, 218
apoptosis, 84, 115, 116, 182, 183, 184, 185, 186, 193, 194
apoptotic pathways, 186
appraisals, 133, 144
arousal, 4, 18, 30, 38, 227
arrhythmogenic, 219
Arrhythmogenic Right Ventricular Cardiomyopathy, xiv, 218, 220
arteriovenous malformation, 226
arthritis, 133, 137, 145, 146, 153, 165, 176, 199
arthroscopic debridement, 169
arthroscopy, viii, xii, 150, 159, 163, 169, 171, 172
ascites, 175, 177, 179, 181
Asian Americans, v, vii, ix, 47, 48, 60, 79, 82

asymptomatic, 156, 158
athletes, 155, 159, 168
atrial myxoma, xiv, 218
atrophy, xv, 104, 110, 229, 233, 235, 236
attachment and its role in medical care, vi, 119
attachment and medical care, 124
attachment style, 129
attachment system, xi, 120, 122, 123, 124, 126, 130, 136
attachment theory, xi, 119, 120, 121, 124, 125, 135, 136, 141
attitudes, 58, 69, 70, 80
autoantibodies, 134
autoimmune disease, xii, 133, 174, 181, 192
autoimmune lymphoproliferative syndrome, xii, 174, 175, 176, 183, 193, 194, 195
autoimmunity, 183, 185, 186, 195
autonomy, 125, 126
autophagy, x, 84, 92, 100, 101, 107, 108, 111, 115, 116
autopsy, 219, 221
autosomal recessive, 100
avascular necrosis, 153
avoidance, 33, 54, 127, 136
awareness, 54, 72, 76, 80, 82

B

bacteria, xiii, 198, 202, 203, 204, 206, 207, 212, 213
bacterium, 213, 214
barriers, vii, x, 48, 50, 58, 63, 65, 68, 73, 74, 76
basal ganglia, 230, 233
base, 88, 89, 121, 123, 138, 146, 164
basic research, 75
behavioral change, 37
behavioral medicine, 141

behaviors, vii, 15, 18, 24, 26, 49, 50, 51, 52, 53, 55, 57, 59, 63, 65, 67, 68, 73, 77, 78, 80, 115, 120, 121, 124, 146
beneficial effect, 208
bilateral, xv, 154, 166, 171, 218
biochemical action, 13
biochemistry, 104
biodiversity, xiii, 198, 205
biopsy, 185, 207, 212
biosynthesis, 8, 14, 117
bleeding, 199, 222
blood, xv, 26, 52, 110, 134, 162, 218, 222, 223
blood flow, 162
blood pressure, 223
body size, 21, 39
body weight, 28
bonding, 124, 126
bone, 154, 158, 163, 164, 166, 176, 177, 178, 179
bone marrow, 176, 177, 178
bowel, viii, xiii, 132, 197, 209, 210
bradycardia, xiv, 217
brain, ix, x, 2, 3, 4, 5, 6, 7, 9, 11, 15, 16, 18, 19, 20, 21, 22, 25, 28, 30, 34, 37, 42, 83, 85, 95, 108, 223, 234
brainstem, 223, 227
bronchospasm, xv, 218, 223

C

calcium, 84, 105
caloric restriction, 114
campaigns, 76, 77
Cancer, 36, 86, 116, 130, 132, 139, 142, 144, 145, 187, 188
capsule, 150, 151, 155, 159, 166, 172
carbohydrate, 4, 6, 10, 11, 21, 26, 28, 31, 202, 226
cardiac arrest, viii, xiv, xv, 217, 218, 219, 222, 223, 225

Index

cardiac muscle, 221
cardiac tamponade, xiv, 218, 221, 222
cardiomyopathies, 219
cardiomyopathy, xiv, 218, 225
cardiovascular disease, 129, 130
caregivers, 135, 142, 147
cartilage, 155, 161, 162, 163
caspase-8, 193
catalytic activity, 14
catecholaminergic polymorphic ventricular tachycardia (CPVT), 219, 225
catecholamines, 6, 14, 43
CD95, 182
CDC, 48, 49, 50, 58
cell biology, 104
cell culture, 91
cell cycle, 95
cell death, 193
cell line, x, 33, 84, 85, 91, 94, 102, 108
cell surface, 16, 25, 186
central nervous system, ix, 2, 3, 28
cerebral palsy, 156, 157, 169
challenges, 20, 50, 56, 102, 108, 133, 211
changing environment, 39
child development, 143
childhood, 32, 143, 147, 202
children, 52, 65, 67, 74, 120, 121, 122, 123, 140, 153, 156, 157, 158, 169
Chronic Diseases, 129, 130
chronic fatigue syndrome, 115
chronic illness, 136
chronic kidney disease, 129, 142, 143
chronic kidney failure, 134
classification, 152, 193
cleavage, 94, 96, 97, 98, 99, 103
cleavage-stimulated mtDNA degradation, 94
clients, 71, 77
clinical interventions, vii, xi, 120
clinical presentation, 168, 182, 184, 192
closed reduction, 162, 163, 170

clustered regularly interspaced short palindromic repeats (CRISPR), x, 84, 86, 99, 106
coding, 59, 84, 94
cognitive dysfunction, 136
cognitive reaction, 144
colitis, 199, 206, 210, 213, 214, 215
collaboration, 57, 131, 140
college students, 52, 73, 81
colorectal cancer, xiii, 198
communication, 52, 72, 80, 129, 140, 147, 204
community, xiii, 48, 51, 52, 53, 54, 55, 57, 59, 74, 75, 76, 80, 81, 198, 205, 208, 209, 230
community service, 59
compensating effect, 93
complex carbohydrates, 202, 211
complex interactions, 10
complexity, 3, 13, 16, 91, 97, 128, 201, 203, 204, 208
compliance, 128, 134, 135, 138, 141
complications, viii, xv, 131, 153, 159, 161, 169, 181, 199, 218, 222, 229, 234
composition, viii, xiii, xiv, 103, 198, 201, 202, 203, 205, 207, 208, 212
compounds, ix, 2, 6, 30
concordance, 141, 200
conduction, 219, 220
connective tissue, 154, 158, 181, 192
consensus, xii, 3, 59, 71, 174, 175, 177, 179, 182, 187, 189
conservation, 10, 17
constituents, 207
consumption, 136, 139
content analysis, 59, 97
controlled trials, 208, 231
controversial, xi, xii, 149, 150, 164, 166
conversations, 52, 67, 69, 71, 75
coronary arteries, 221, 225
coronary artery bypass graft, 145
coronary artery disease, 225

correlation, vii, xiv, 184, 198, 203
cost, 131, 136, 140
counseling, 111, 137, 140, 145, 146
creatinine, 135
cross-sectional study, 81, 138
CT scan, 155, 162
cultural beliefs, 50
cultural norms, 54, 59, 67, 74
culture, x, 48, 51, 53, 55, 67, 70, 71, 74, 75
cytochrome, 13, 99
cytokines, 183, 207
cytoplasm, 14
cytosine, 88

D

daily treatment, 102
data collection, 57, 58, 59, 75
deaths, 108, 130, 226
decision-making process, 45, 128
defects, x, 26, 84, 85, 182, 186
deficiency, 17, 18, 157, 162, 193
deficit, 18, 23, 165
degenerative arthritis, 156
degenerative joint disease, 161
degradation, 23, 94, 96, 101, 106, 202, 211
delayed testing, 50
depressive symptoms, 147
deprivation, 15, 17, 18, 23
depth, 57, 74, 150
desiccation, viii, 2, 4, 21
diabetes, ix, 2, 3, 7, 20, 29, 35, 44, 86, 103, 105, 113, 120, 130, 131, 139, 140, 142, 185
diagnostic criteria, xii, 174, 175, 177, 178, 179, 182, 184, 185, 187, 189, 191, 193
diet, xiii, 10, 25, 30, 131, 198, 201, 203, 211
dietary fiber, 203, 207
dietary regimes, 10
differential diagnosis, 182
digestive enzymes, 202

digestive haemorrhage, 222
dilatative, xiv, 218, 219
dimerization, 97, 98
disability, 130, 133, 232
disclosure, 54, 59, 73, 74
discomfort, 74, 130, 135, 152
discrimination, 54, 55, 56, 76, 81, 82
disease activity, 137, 202
disease gene, 213
disease model, 99
disease progression, 87
diseases, vii, x, xii, xiv, 18, 27, 28, 40, 83, 84, 85, 86, 87, 93, 96, 97, 100, 101, 102, 106, 108, 111, 112, 114, 115, 116, 117, 130, 132, 141, 144, 147, 156, 174, 177, 178, 181, 187, 217, 218, 219, 222, 223
dislocation, vii, xi, xii, 149, 150, 151, 152, 153, 154, 155, 156, 159, 160, 161, 162, 163, 164, 165, 166, 167, 168, 169, 170, 171
disorder, xiii, xiv, 18, 90, 104, 117, 158, 174, 178, 179, 182, 184, 193, 197, 200, 217, 219, 233
dissociation, xiv, 218, 222
distress, 81, 130, 132
distribution, 38, 199, 200
diversity, 19, 125, 200, 205, 208, 212, 215
DNA, v, x, xiii, 42, 83, 85, 86, 88, 89, 95, 96, 97, 99, 103, 104, 105, 106, 108, 110, 111, 112, 116, 188, 189, 198, 205
DNA damage, 42, 111
DNA polymerase, 89
DNA sequencing, xiii, 198, 205
dopamine, viii, ix, xv, 2, 3, 4, 15, 24, 29, 30, 31, 34, 35, 36, 37, 39, 40, 43, 45, 229, 230, 234
dopaminergic, 14, 18, 24, 25, 31, 230, 234
Down syndrome, 154, 156, 158, 169
down-regulation, 207
Drosophila, 4, 5, 6, 7, 8, 10, 12, 14, 15, 16, 17, 18, 20, 21, 22, 24, 25, 26, 27, 28, 30,

Index

31, 32, 33, 34, 35, 36, 37, 38, 39, 40, 41, 42, 43, 44, 45, 110
drug therapy, 202
drug treatment, xiii, 198
drugs, 45, 49, 67, 68, 69, 70, 91, 102, 128, 205, 219, 231
dualism, 226
dysplasia, xi, xii, 149, 150, 151, 156, 157, 158, 159, 162, 165, 168, 169, 170, 171

E

E. coli, 207
East Asia, 51, 53, 74
eating disorders, 27
Ecological Systems Theory, 51
ecology, 79, 121, 208
economic status, 129
education, 49, 60, 65, 68, 72, 77, 123, 137, 140, 145, 146
effects of rapamycin, 102
effusion, 188, 192
Ehlers-Danlos syndrome, 154
embolism, xv, 218, 221, 222
embryogenesis, 89, 113
empathy, 122, 123, 125
encoding, 5, 8, 13, 21, 24, 39, 42
endocrine, x, 4, 5, 10, 13, 22, 28, 31, 43, 83, 85, 87, 226, 227
endonuclease, 94, 100, 103, 107, 111
endothelial cells, 178, 184
energy, vii, viii, xi, 2, 3, 4, 5, 6, 8, 11, 15, 17, 18, 19, 26, 27, 28, 34, 40, 44, 87, 149, 150, 153, 154, 155, 164, 167, 202, 203, 207, 211
energy expenditure, 3, 40
energy homeostasis, viii, 2, 3, 4, 5, 6, 11, 18, 26, 27, 28, 34
environment, viii, 2, 17, 19, 27, 51, 121, 126, 159, 200, 210
environmental conditions, 3

environmental factors, 33, 199, 200, 201
environmental influences, 209
environmental stimuli, 33
environmental stress, viii, 2, 4, 20, 23
enzymes, 13, 14, 21, 23, 24, 28, 85, 94, 95, 99, 101, 202
epidemiology, 139, 209
epithelial cells, 203, 204, 207
epithelium, 203, 204, 205, 208
Epstein-Barr virus, 178
equilibrium, 3, 92, 202
ethnic groups, 48, 49, 56, 137
etiology, 20, 130, 154, 175, 177, 187
everolimus, 102
evidence, viii, xii, xiii, xiv, 13, 15, 21, 22, 90, 107, 133, 140, 154, 164, 165, 174, 175, 177, 178, 179, 184, 187, 189, 198, 200, 206
evolution, ix, 2, 3, 7, 12, 14, 15, 35, 45, 84, 104, 130, 201, 210, 223
exclusion, 58, 177, 179, 184, 187, 213
expertise, 125, 132
exposure, 63, 68, 200, 226
extra-uterine pregnancy rupture, 222
extrusion, 162

F

facilitators, vii, 50, 58, 65
families, 4, 52, 54, 60, 74, 80, 139, 140
family environment, 65
family members, 54, 55, 63, 70, 73, 74, 186
family relationships, 54, 132
family support, 54, 74
family system, 54
fasting, 10, 44
fat, 5, 8, 9, 11, 15, 17, 21, 22, 25, 26, 27, 30, 33, 35, 37, 40, 203, 227
fatty acids, 107, 203, 207, 211
fear, x, 48, 54, 55, 58, 59, 63, 64, 68, 69, 70, 72, 73, 74, 125, 136, 144

feelings, 68, 72, 126
femur, 151, 154, 157, 161, 165, 166
fermentation, 203
fever, viii, xii, 173, 175, 177, 184, 185, 199
fiber content, 203
fibers, 96, 203, 221
fibroblasts, 114, 184
fibrosis, 177, 178, 180
fluctuations, 3, 235
follicles, 174, 175
food, 3, 16, 17, 18, 28
food intake, 17, 18
force, 151, 153, 162
fractures, 151, 152, 161, 162, 167
frontal cortex, 29
full capacity, 134
fulminant hepatitis, 223
functional analysis, 41
fungi, 204, 206
fusion, 92, 104

G

gait, 156, 233
gastrectomy, 144
gastrointestinal tract, 199, 202, 211
gene expression, 23, 24, 33, 39, 41, 97, 109, 206, 213
gene regulation, 15, 105
gene therapy, 97, 102
gene transfer, 108
general anesthesia, 162
generalizability, 78
genes, 8, 11, 13, 14, 18, 23, 24, 27, 28, 37, 40, 45, 84, 91, 100, 103, 182, 184, 189, 202
genetic defect, 182
genetic disease, 108
genetic drift, 91
genetic information, 107
genetic therapy, 94

genetics, xiii, 33, 111, 198, 225
genome, x, 84, 85, 87, 88, 89, 90, 99, 103, 107, 110, 111, 147
glomerulonephritis, 192
glucagon, ix, 2, 4, 5, 11, 26, 31, 32, 42
glucose, 5, 9, 18, 21, 26, 29, 37, 101, 103, 203, 214
glucose tolerance, 102
GnRH, 12
goblet cells, 204
gonadotropin-releasing hormone, 36
growth, 4, 7, 8, 15, 20, 22, 26, 30, 32, 33, 35, 36, 37, 39, 40, 41, 42, 44, 48, 156, 203
growth factor, 4, 36
growth rate, 48
guilty, 114
gut microbiota, xiii, 198, 200, 202, 206, 207, 208, 210, 211, 212, 213, 214

H

haemorrhage, xiv, xv, 218, 222
haplotypes, 90, 95
health care, xi, 50, 54, 77, 81, 120, 125, 126, 127, 131, 132, 136, 139, 144, 145
health care system, 127
health promotion, 147
health psychology, 138, 142, 146
health services, 127, 136, 146
health status, 81
heart block, 221
heart disease, 107, 225
hegemony, 55
hemoglobinopathies, 130
hemolytic anemia, 183
hemopericardium, xiv, 218, 221
hemorrhage, 224
hepatomegaly, 179
herpes, xii, 109, 173, 175, 178, 188
herpes simplex, 109

herpes virus, xii, 173, 175, 178, 188
heterogeneity, 87, 102, 130
heteroplasmy, vii, x, 84, 85, 86, 87, 88, 89, 90, 91, 92, 93, 94, 95, 96, 97, 101, 102, 103, 106, 107, 109, 110, 111, 112
HHV-8, xii, 173, 174, 175, 176, 177, 178, 183, 184, 187, 188, 189, 190
hip arthroplasty, 165
hip disloaction, 150
hip joint, 150, 153, 154, 156, 167
hip replacement, xii, 150, 171
histamine, xv, 218
HIV knowledge, 51, 53, 57, 65, 66, 73, 75
HIV test, vii, ix, 48, 49, 50, 51, 52, 53, 54, 55, 56, 57, 63, 65, 66, 68, 69, 72, 73, 74, 76, 77, 78, 80, 81, 82
HIV testing behaviors among AAPI, 50
HIV/AIDS, v, vii, ix, xii, 47, 48, 49, 50, 51, 52, 53, 54, 55, 56, 57, 58, 59, 63, 64, 65, 66, 67, 68, 69, 70, 71, 72, 73, 74, 75, 76, 77, 78, 79, 80, 81, 82, 141, 173, 175, 176, 187, 188, 189, 194
HIV-related stigma, 50, 55, 57, 69, 73, 74, 75, 76, 82
homeostasis, vii, viii, 2, 3, 4, 5, 6, 7, 8, 11, 14, 17, 18, 19, 21, 26, 27, 28, 31, 33, 34, 37, 38, 40, 41, 43, 84, 92, 93, 103, 186, 195, 203, 208
homosexuality, 50, 54, 55, 65, 74
hopelessness, 127, 136
hormone, 3, 5, 11, 12, 17, 18, 23, 25, 28, 31, 34, 36, 38, 39, 41, 42, 43, 44
hospitalization, 126, 128, 140
host, 8, 102, 202, 203, 204, 206, 207, 210, 211, 215
human behavior, 147
human brain, 104
human condition, xiii, 198
human development, 51, 79, 138
human genome, 100
human health, 213
human motivation, 143

Hunter, 124, 126, 130, 141, 143, 144, 145, 213
hyaline, 174, 175, 176, 177, 181
hydrogen, 24, 207
hydrogen peroxide, 24
hydrolysis, 89
hydrops, 227
hyperactivity, 17, 18, 38
hypergammaglobulinemia, 178, 181, 183
hyperhidrosis, 180
hyperplasia, 175, 186, 187, 188, 191, 192
hypertension, 222
hypertrichosis, 180
hypertrophic, xiv, 218, 219
hypertrophic cardiomyopathy, xiv, 218
hypertrophy, xiv, 218
hypoglycemia, 26
hypothalamus, 27
hypothesis, 88, 93, 100, 151, 153
hypoxia, xv, 218

I

iatrogenic, xi, 149, 159, 160, 161, 166, 169
IBD, xiii, xiv, 132, 133, 197, 198, 199, 200, 201, 202, 204, 205, 206, 207, 208, 209, 210
identical twins, 212
identification, 21, 28, 43, 54, 57
idiopathic, xii, 156, 174, 175, 178, 189, 190, 191, 192, 193, 199, 233
IL-6, 174, 177, 178, 179, 180, 181, 184, 185, 189, 194
ileum, 199, 202
iliopsoas, 151, 159
illicit drug use, 141
illness care, 143
imbalances, 205, 212, 214
immigrants, 50, 53, 56, 81
immigration, 56, 77
immune defense, 14

immune modulation, 212
immune response, 13
immune system, xiii, 102, 103, 193, 198, 200, 205, 206
immunity, 210
immunobiology, 210
immunogenicity, 102
immunoglobulin, 183
immunosuppression, 101
improvements, xiii, 127, 159, 198, 205
in vitro, 99, 186, 230
in vivo, 29, 33, 99, 108, 211
incidence, 151, 152, 153, 157, 168, 181, 199, 200, 210
individual development, 51
individual differences, 124
individuals, 48, 49, 50, 54, 55, 58, 60, 63, 65, 71, 73, 74, 76, 87, 90, 112, 122, 126, 131, 132, 136, 208
induction, 9, 195, 213
infection, viii, 2, 4, 49, 53, 54, 55, 65, 66, 73, 79, 175, 177, 188, 206, 209, 227
inflammasome, 114, 115, 116, 117
inflammation, xiii, 36, 113, 133, 198, 199, 203, 206, 207, 208, 213, 220
Inflammatory Bowel Disease, viii, 132, 137, 198, 209, 210, 211, 212, 214, 215
inflammatory disease, 199
inflammatory responses, 177
influenza, 230
inheritance, 89, 110
inhibition, 11, 13, 15, 33, 117
initiation, 30, 201
innate immunity, 208
insects, vii, viii, 2, 4, 6, 9, 11, 13, 14, 15, 19, 21, 22, 28, 31, 34, 37, 38, 44
insulin, ix, 2, 3, 4, 5, 7, 8, 10, 16, 20, 21, 22, 25, 26, 27, 30, 32, 33, 34, 35, 36, 37, 38, 39, 40, 41, 42, 43, 44
insulin resistance, 20, 36
insulin signaling, 4, 8, 20, 21, 22, 27, 35, 37, 39, 44

insulin-like peptides, ix, 2, 3, 4, 32, 35, 37, 42, 44
integration, 73, 102
intercourse, 49, 52
interdependence, 74
intermittent dosing, 101
internal mechanisms, 27
internal working models, 123, 138
internalized HIV/AIDS stigma, 51
interpersonal relations, 120, 132, 133
interpersonal relationships, 120, 132, 133
intervention, 77, 78, 127, 138, 140, 209
intestinal malabsorption, 199
intestine, 7, 202, 203, 204, 211, 213
intimacy, 122, 123, 145
intracranial pressure, xv, 218, 223
irritable bowel syndrome, 215
ischemia, xiv, 217
ischemic attack, 223
issues, vii, 49, 54, 65, 74, 82, 108, 124
Italy, 119, 149, 210, 217, 226

J

Japan, 61, 173, 177
joint pain, 133
joints, 150, 158

K

Kidney Disease, 134
kidney failure, 134
kidney transplantation, 134
kinetics, 95

L

Lactobacillus, 207, 213
larvae, 5, 7, 12, 16, 18, 23, 27, 30
larval stages, 8

latency, 129, 178
leakage, 88, 89, 108
left ventricle, 219
lesions, 111, 174, 175, 179, 180, 191
levodopa induced dyskinesias, 232
ligament, 150, 151, 155, 166, 167
ligand, 9, 12, 183, 186
light, 27, 49, 187
lipid metabolism, 4, 28, 44
lipids, 11, 203
liver, x, 11, 27, 44, 83, 85, 136, 199
localization, 38, 44, 88, 94, 96, 98
locomotor, 4, 17, 18, 26, 41
loneliness, 145, 146
longevity, 10, 20, 24, 34
longitudinal study, 81
lumen, 203, 204
lung cancer, 109, 117, 191
lung disease, 185, 191
Luo, 39, 40, 110
Lupus, 133, 134, 137, 147, 192
lupus erythematosus, 133, 137
lymph node, viii, xii, 173, 174, 175, 176, 177, 178, 180, 184, 185, 186, 187, 188, 191, 192
lymphadenopathy, xiii, 174, 175, 176, 178, 179, 180, 181, 182, 183, 185, 193
lymphocytes, 183, 185
lymphoid tissue, 174
lymphoma, xii, 174, 176, 178, 188, 189, 219
lysine, 106

M

macrophages, 204
magnetic resonance, 162
magnetic resonance imaging, 162
majority, 16, 64, 65, 182, 206
malignancy, xii, 173, 212
mammals, ix, 2, 4, 5, 9, 10, 11, 14, 16, 21, 22, 26, 27, 33, 210
management, xi, 120, 130, 131, 133, 135, 138, 141, 142, 159, 163, 164, 167, 171, 190, 209, 215, 225
manipulation, 18, 25, 99
mass, viii, xii, 33, 173
massive pulmonary bleeding, 222
maternal lineage, 87
mechanical stress, 22
media, 16, 67, 68, 72
medical, vii, xi, xiv, 50, 55, 64, 120, 124, 126, 127, 128, 129, 130, 131, 132, 135, 136, 142, 143, 144, 146, 151, 198, 225
medical care, vii, xi, 50, 120, 124, 130, 142
medical science, 144
medication, 128, 129, 137, 138, 140, 141, 143, 145, 146
medication compliance, 137
medicine, 137, 141, 143, 145, 168, 215, 225
mellitus, 86, 105
memory, 14, 128, 195
mental health, 67, 135
mental model, 126, 135
mental representation, 121
meta-analysis, 137, 147, 208, 214
metabolic disorders, ix, 2, 11, 29, 36, 200, 209
metabolic pathways, ix, 2, 203
metabolism, vii, ix, 2, 3, 4, 5, 6, 7, 8, 15, 18, 22, 23, 26, 27, 28, 30, 32, 34, 35, 39, 40, 41, 44, 203, 211, 214
metamorphosis, 8, 14
mice, 18, 20, 28, 43, 95, 186, 195, 206, 213, 214
microbial community, 202, 212
microbiota, viii, xiii, xiv, 198, 200, 201, 202, 203, 204, 205, 206, 207, 208, 209, 210, 211, 212, 213, 214, 215
microorganisms, xiii, 198, 204
midbrain, 18, 25
mitochondria, 84, 88, 89, 90, 92, 93, 94, 95, 96, 98, 99, 100, 101, 102, 103, 104, 108, 109, 110, 111, 116

mitochondrial disorders, 90
mitochondrial DNA, x, 84, 89, 91, 103, 104, 105, 106, 107, 108, 109, 110, 111, 112, 115
mitochondrial genome, 85, 87, 88, 89, 90, 92, 94, 98, 99, 103, 106, 107
mitochondrial heteroplasmy, 87, 90, 110, 112
mitochondrial mutation, 91, 93, 94, 107, 110
mitochondria-targeted enzyme, 94
mitotypes, 88, 90
model system, vii, ix, 2, 7, 22, 39
models, x, xi, 20, 76, 78, 84, 92, 93, 95, 96, 98, 99, 102, 105, 120, 121, 126
moderates, 126, 135, 145
modifications, 37, 111
molecules, 90, 91, 92, 93, 203, 204
mollusks, 12
monomers, 96, 97, 98
monozygotic twins, 200, 205
morbidity, 131, 134, 156
morphogenesis, 37
morphology, 154, 157
mortality, 30, 124, 129, 130, 131, 134
mosquitoes, 64
motivation, 14, 26, 29, 50, 69, 121
motor behavior, 24
motor neurons, 13
mRNA, 25, 34, 97
mtDNA, vii, x, 84, 85, 86, 87, 88, 89, 90, 91, 92, 93, 94, 95, 96, 97, 98, 99, 100, 101, 102, 103, 104, 106, 107, 108, 109, 110, 111, 112
    disorders, 94
    genome, 90, 92
mTORC1, 101
mucosa, 199, 206, 207, 213, 214
mucus, 204, 208, 215
Multicentric Castleman's disease, viii, xii, 173, 174, 176, 178, 190
multi-ethnic, 80

multiple rearranged mtDNAs, 90
muscles, 9, 33, 87, 150, 158
musculoskeletal, 130
mutagenesis, 5, 41
mutant, vii, x, 18, 84, 85, 87, 91, 92, 93, 94, 96, 97, 99, 100, 101, 102, 103, 106, 108, 109, 195
mutant alleles, 93
mutant mtDNA, vii, x, 84, 87, 91, 92, 94, 96, 97, 99, 100, 101, 102, 108
mutation, 18, 87, 88, 91, 92, 94, 96, 98, 101, 102, 103, 105, 106, 108, 110, 111, 116, 183, 185, 193, 194
mutation rate, 87
mutations, vii, x, 17, 20, 21, 24, 83, 85, 87, 88, 89, 90, 91, 93, 95, 96, 99, 100, 102, 104, 105, 106, 107, 109, 110, 182, 193
myoblasts, 106
myocardial infarction, 225
myocarditis, xiv, 218, 219
myocardium, 219
myopathy, 90, 115

N

nanoparticles, 116
narratives, 65, 77, 145
necrosis, 167, 227
necrotizing acute pancreatitis, 223
negative emotions, 135
nerve, 8, 9, 151, 153, 230
nervous system, 15, 28, 40, 87
neurodegeneration, 93
neurodegenerative diseases, 11, 29
neurodegenerative disorders, 7, 233
neuroendocrine cells, 37
neurons, 6, 8, 14, 16, 19, 21, 24, 25, 30, 31, 33, 39, 41, 230
neuropathy, 94, 96, 131, 181
neuropeptides, ix, 2, 4, 11, 13
neurophysiology, 7, 42

neurosecretory, 5, 7, 19
neurotransmitter, ix, 2, 4, 18, 39
neurotransmitters, ix, 2, 4, 6
neutral, 64, 91
neutropenia, 183
new HIV diagnosis, 48
NMDA receptors, 230
nodes, 184, 186
nodules, 185, 186
North America, 165, 199
nuclear genome, 87, 88, 97
nucleus, 23, 29, 84, 98, 103, 227
nutrient, 5, 7, 15, 16, 19, 21, 22, 23, 25, 27, 28, 30, 33, 36, 39, 40, 42, 43, 101, 201, 202, 203, 204, 211
nutrition, 10, 22, 27, 211
nutritional status, 9, 26

O

obesity, ix, 2, 3, 7, 17, 27, 29, 30, 32, 34, 36
oedema, 223
optic nerve, x, 83, 85
optimism, 209
oral hypoglycemic medications, 131
organ, 9, 11, 19, 23, 27, 28, 83, 85, 87, 129, 130, 138, 202, 203, 211
organelles, 84, 91, 92, 105, 112
organism, viii, 2, 3, 4, 9, 19, 22, 26, 27, 33, 44, 51, 86
ossification, 153
osteoarthritis, 153, 156, 166, 168, 171
Osteogenesis, 154, 156
osteotomy, xi, 150, 160, 164, 165, 168, 170, 171
overlap, 182, 186, 233
oxidation, 84
oxidative damage, 88, 107
oxidative stress, 5, 13, 22, 31, 34, 36, 38, 44, 207
OXPHOS function, 94, 96

P

p53, 20
Pacific, v, vii, ix, 47, 48, 60, 61, 78, 79, 80, 81, 82
Pacific Islanders, vii, ix, 48, 60, 79, 81, 82
pain, 114, 127, 130, 133, 136, 139, 144, 156, 164, 166, 199
pain perception, 136, 139
pancreatitis, 223, 227
paraneoplastic syndrome, 179
parents, 52, 65, 66, 67, 71, 72, 74, 103
Parkin, x, 84, 85, 93, 100, 108, 111
participants, 52, 57, 58, 63, 64, 65, 66, 67, 68, 69, 70, 72, 73, 74, 76, 78
pathogenesis, xiii, 177, 179, 183, 184, 189, 198, 200, 205, 210, 225, 226, 234
pathogens, xiii, 198, 203, 204, 206
pathology, 93, 163, 226
pathophysiological roles, 105
pathophysiology, 187, 225, 227
pathway, 4, 6, 7, 8, 13, 16, 20, 22, 23, 26, 30, 31, 32, 33, 37, 41, 113, 186, 189, 219
pedal, 151, 166
pelvis, 152, 161, 171
pemphigus, 181, 192
peptides, ix, 2, 3, 4, 5, 8, 12, 13, 30, 31, 32, 35, 37, 38, 42, 44, 204
perceived health, 130
pericarditis, 221
pericardium, xiv, 218
peripheral nervous system, 234
peripheral neuropathy, 179
peripheral vascular disease, 131
permeability, 203, 205
personality, 134, 140, 141, 146
pH, 203
phage, 206, 214
pharmaceutical, 208
pharmacological treatment, 219
pharmacotherapy, 129, 135

phenotypes, viii, x, xiv, 8, 20, 41, 84, 85, 182, 198, 200, 206, 213
phosphorus, 142
phosphorylation, x, 9, 11, 14, 30, 44, 84, 85, 114
phosphorylation events, 9
phylum, 204, 205
physicians, xi, 120, 141
physiological mechanisms, 3, 28
physiology, ix, 2, 4, 33, 107
plasma cells, 175, 178, 179, 180, 184, 185, 186
pleural effusion, 175, 179, 181
pneumothorax, xv, 218, 222
point mutation, 87, 88, 89, 96, 106
policy, 75, 76
polycythemia, 180
polymerase, 89, 91
polymorphism, 184, 194
population, ix, 11, 48, 49, 51, 53, 56, 57, 71, 75, 78, 81, 82, 86, 87, 91, 93, 104, 109, 130, 131, 156, 165, 200
population group, 51
population size, 78, 104
positive correlation, 134
positive relationship, 130
positive status, 63, 69, 73
post-traumatic stress disorder, 129
potassium, 219
Practice implications, 77
predictive validity, 147
prefrontal cortex, 33
pregnancy, 53, 222
premature death, 130
prevention, 49, 50, 52, 58, 66, 76, 77, 78, 80, 82, 129
probiotics, 204, 209
professionals, 77, 128, 135, 136, 139
prognosis, 153, 174
programming, 10, 33
progressive supranuclear palsy, xv, 229, 233, 235

proliferation, 158, 174, 178, 182, 186
protection, 22, 54, 120, 121
protein sequence, 98
protein synthesis, 9
proteins, x, 21, 22, 84, 85, 92, 93, 97, 100, 109, 202, 204
psychiatry, 136, 141, 143
psychoanalysis, 120
psychological distress, 55, 74, 132
psychological processes, xi, 120, 126
psychological variables, 129
psychological well-being, 124, 132
psychosocial factors, 132
psychosomatic, 124, 139, 145
psychotherapy, 139
public health, ix, 2, 3, 78, 125, 141
pulmonary artery, xv, 218
pulmonary hypertension, 180, 222
pulmonary vascular resistance, xv, 218
pulmonary venous thrombo-embolism, 222
punishment, 65

Q

quality control, 92, 100
quality of life, vii, xi, 120, 132, 133, 134, 135, 136, 137, 138, 142
questionnaire, 58, 64, 73

R

Rapamycin, 101, 105
  analogs, 102
  treatment, 102, 103
reactions, 19, 22, 121
reactive oxygen, 21, 24, 88, 109
receptor, viii, xv, 8, 12, 15, 16, 17, 20, 25, 27, 32, 34, 36, 41, 184, 186, 190, 194, 227, 229, 230, 234
recognition, 68, 74, 94, 95, 108, 177, 204
recombination, 90, 100, 104, 107, 109, 111

Index

recommendations, iv, 76, 128
reconstruction, 166, 170, 172
recovery, 159, 207, 209, 214
rectus femoris, 150, 167
relational dimension, 130, 135
relational model, xi, 56, 119
relevance, 124, 131, 145
remission, 207, 212, 214
repair, 88, 111, 164, 166
replication, 88, 89, 91, 92, 93, 104, 107, 175
reproduction, 5, 8, 44
requirement, viii, 2, 87, 96, 177
researchers, 50, 52, 59, 76, 122
resilience, 201, 210, 214
resistance, xv, 5, 7, 8, 13, 19, 21, 24, 26, 32, 34, 38, 42, 44, 184, 206, 214, 218, 223
resources, 15, 127
respiratory failure, xv, 218
response, viii, xiv, 2, 4, 6, 10, 13, 15, 16, 17, 18, 19, 21, 22, 24, 26, 27, 30, 35, 36, 92, 130, 184, 189, 198, 205, 208, 231, 232, 234
responsiveness, 26, 125, 137, 147
restoration, 94, 114
restriction enzyme (RE), 94, 95
restrictive, xiv, 180, 218, 219
restrictive cardiomyopathy, xiv, 218
restrictive lung disease, 180
retina, x, 83, 85
retinitis pigmentosa, 94
rheumatoid arthritis, 181, 192
rhythm, xiv, 217, 219, 221
ribosomal RNA, 84
right ventricle, 222
risk, vii, x, xiii, 48, 49, 50, 51, 52, 53, 54, 55, 57, 58, 63, 65, 68, 71, 73, 75, 76, 77, 78, 79, 80, 81, 82, 129, 131, 142, 143, 146, 153, 161, 162, 187, 190, 198, 200, 201, 202, 207, 208, 215, 225, 226
risk factors, 49, 68, 79, 143, 161, 226
RNA, 43, 99, 106

S

S6K, 9
safety, 122, 125, 165
sarcoidosis, 219, 220
science, 141, 145
secrete, 8, 16, 25, 35
secretion, ix, 2, 4, 5, 9, 16, 19, 30, 35, 40, 41, 43, 194, 204
segregation, 91, 104, 108, 109
self-efficacy, 53, 138
self-fertilization, 104
self-regulation, xi, 120, 126, 127
senescence, 6, 24, 31, 40, 107
sensing, 5, 7, 15, 21, 26, 28, 37, 40
sensitivity, 18, 28, 42
sequencing, 89, 107, 206, 210, 215
serum, 178, 180, 181, 183, 184
service provider, 56, 64, 77
services, 50, 55, 56, 57, 72, 80, 82, 128
sex, 49, 50, 52, 53, 54, 63, 64, 65, 66, 67, 68, 69, 70, 71, 74, 76, 79, 80
sexual behavior, 52, 53, 54, 55, 65, 73, 74, 81
sexual health, 53, 67, 72, 75
sexual orientation, 54, 56, 61, 65, 74
sexuality, 55, 65, 67, 68, 71, 72, 74
sexually transmitted infections, 72
side effects, 97, 101, 233
signal transduction, 8, 20, 26
signaling pathway, 5, 16, 19, 22
signalling, 30, 35, 37, 41
signals, 9, 21, 27, 33, 43, 92, 98, 127, 213
skeletal muscle, 90, 104, 112
skin, 113, 130, 176, 179, 180
SLE, 133, 134, 178
slipped capital femoral epiphysis, 161
small intestine, 199, 202
smoking, xiii, 198, 200, 201
social change, 77
social desirability, 78

social development, 120
social interaction, 131, 132
social network, 51, 57, 59, 69
social psychology, 140, 141, 146
social relations, 132
social relationships, 132
social services, 57
social support, 53, 69, 129, 132, 133, 144
social workers, 77
society, 76, 139, 143
socioeconomic status, 200
sodium, 206, 213, 219
South Asia, 74, 79, 80, 82
Southeast Asia, 52, 74, 80
Spain, 83, 112, 113, 197, 210
species, 7, 11, 15, 21, 24, 88, 109, 202, 205, 206, 207, 208, 211
species richness, 205
splenomegaly, 175, 179, 182, 183
stability, 100, 104, 108, 121, 150, 154, 159, 161, 163, 167, 201, 210
starvation, 5, 8, 13, 16, 17, 18, 22, 25, 26, 27, 28, 38, 42
state, xiii, 9, 15, 42, 48, 76, 85, 90, 98, 107, 136, 177, 198, 223
stigma, x, 48, 50, 51, 54, 55, 57, 64, 69, 70, 71, 72, 73, 74, 75, 76, 77, 78, 81, 82
stigmatized, 54, 76, 78
stillbirth, 226, 227
stimulation, 13, 15, 19, 207
storage, 3, 8, 26, 27, 28, 35
stratification, 190
stress, vii, viii, 2, 3, 4, 6, 7, 8, 13, 16, 19, 20, 21, 22, 25, 29, 30, 31, 32, 34, 35, 36, 41, 42, 106, 113, 120, 124, 133, 140, 157, 200, 202, 225
stress reactions, 23
stress response, 5, 6, 7, 13, 22, 30, 31, 124
stressful events, 144
stressors, viii, xi, 2, 4, 6, 120, 126, 127, 133
striatum, 14, 25, 29, 37, 43, 147, 234

style, vii, xi, 120, 123, 124, 126, 127, 131, 132, 133, 134, 135, 136, 137, 138, 139, 142, 144, 147
subarachnoid aneurysm, 223
subgroups, 49, 51, 56, 76
sublimons, 90, 107
subluxation, vii, xi, xii, 149, 150, 151, 154, 156, 157, 158, 160, 161, 169, 170
substance abuse, 49, 141
substance use, 67, 81
substrate, 19, 20, 21, 25, 203
sudden death, viii, xiv, 217, 218, 219, 220, 221, 222, 223, 224, 225, 226, 227
sudden infant death syndrome, 227
sulfate, 206, 213
Sun, 105, 138, 188
surgical intervention, 161
surgical resection, 174
surveillance, 48, 49, 79, 82
survival, 3, 10, 15, 16, 17, 25, 32, 120, 130, 165, 166, 195
susceptibility, 31, 51, 53, 59, 130, 213
symptoms, viii, xii, xiv, 102, 116, 127, 132, 133, 136, 146, 158, 160, 165, 173, 175, 177, 178, 180, 199, 217, 231, 232, 233
synapse, 24
synaptic vesicles, 14, 24
syndrome, viii, xii, xiv, 96, 98, 140, 156, 168, 173, 174, 175, 176, 177, 178, 179, 181, 182, 183, 184, 190, 192, 193, 194, 195, 217, 218, 219, 223, 224, 225, 233
synthesis, 14, 23, 24, 31, 36, 37, 107
systemic lupus erythematosus, 137, 181, 191
systemic sclerosis, 181

T

T cell, 182, 183, 184, 185, 186, 193, 195
T cell receptor (TCR), 182, 183

Index

target, 9, 11, 13, 22, 25, 32, 37, 66, 76, 94, 95, 96, 97, 98, 101, 107, 114
target allele, 94
taxa, xiii, 198, 201, 205
TCR, 183, 195
techniques, 89, 159, 162, 168
technology, xiii, 72, 91, 98, 159, 198, 205
temperature, viii, 2, 3, 4
temsirolimus, 102
tendon, 151, 159
tension, xv, 155, 218, 222
tension pneumothorax, xv, 218, 222
tensions, 65
terminally ill, 142
testing, vii, ix, 48, 50, 51, 53, 55, 57, 58, 59, 63, 64, 65, 68, 69, 72, 73, 75, 76, 77, 78
T-helper cell, 184
Theoretical Basis, 121
therapeutic approaches, 205
therapeutics, 215
therapy, viii, xv, 94, 97, 98, 101, 102, 105, 109, 111, 129, 134, 143, 177, 189, 209, 214, 225, 229, 232, 234, 236
Thompson-Epstein, 150, 152
threshold level, x, 84, 85, 93
thrombocytopenia, 177, 183
thrombosis, 221
thymoma, 187
thyroid, 179
tissue, 8, 10, 26, 33, 38, 87, 90, 98, 102, 154, 158, 159, 164, 219
TNF, 177, 184, 204
TNF-α, 184
torsade de pointes, 219
toxic effect, 102
traditional views, 74
traditions, 54, 74
trafficking, 35, 98
transcription, x, 8, 13, 14, 15, 16, 20, 24, 32, 34, 35, 37, 40, 41, 44, 84, 86, 105, 109, 195
transcription factors, 9, 14, 35, 105, 109

transfer RNA, 84
transformation, 102, 186
transition mutation, 89
translation, 9, 30, 101, 106, 154, 155
transmission, 49, 50, 52, 53, 58, 67, 89, 97, 213, 235
transplant, 135, 138, 139
transplant recipients, 135, 138
transplantation, 134, 135, 140, 209, 215
transport, 24, 204, 219
trauma, xi, 123, 149, 150, 151, 153, 154, 166, 167, 169
treatment, vii, ix, x, xi, xii, xiii, xiv, xv, 2, 3, 7, 50, 84, 85, 101, 102, 103, 111, 114, 115, 117, 125, 127, 128, 129, 130, 132, 134, 135, 136, 137, 140, 141, 145, 149, 150, 162, 163, 164, 166, 167, 168, 170, 171, 172, 174, 185, 190, 198, 205, 206, 207, 209, 212, 214, 215, 218, 221, 229, 230, 231, 232, 233, 234, 235
tremor, 230, 231, 232, 233
trial, 140, 141, 235, 236
trisomy 21, 169
tumor, 177, 204
tumor necrosis factor, 177, 204
type 1 diabetes, 139
type 2 diabetes, 131, 140
tyrosine, 14, 18, 23, 40, 41, 43, 143
tyrosine hydroxylase, 14, 18, 23, 40, 41, 43

U

ulcerative colitis, 198, 212, 214
uncleaved mtDNA, 94
United States (USA), 32, 33, 39, 40, 43, 44, 48, 61, 79, 80, 82, 113, 192, 195, 212, 213, 214

V

variables, xi, 60, 62, 63, 120, 126, 135, 144

variations, 15, 106, 125
various levels of stigma, 69
vascular endothelial growth factor (VEGF), 177, 178, 179, 180, 184, 185
vasculitis, 180
vasoconstriction, xv, 218
vasodilation, 222
vector, 95, 97, 98, 151, 163
ventricular fibrillation, xiv, 217, 219, 221, 225
vertebrates, 6, 16, 28, 36
viral infection, 206
viral myocarditis, 221
virus infection, xii, 43, 174, 184
viruses, 204, 206, 213
visualization, 159
vitamin B12, 180, 183
vulnerability, 54, 87, 130, 136

weight loss, viii, xii, 142, 144, 173, 175, 180, 184, 199
Western countries, 181, 199
white death, 219
wild-type mtDNA, vii, x, 84, 85, 92, 93, 94, 95, 96, 100
Wolff-Parkinson-White syndrome, 218, 219, 225
World Health Organization (WHO), 130, 138, 147
worldwide, 131, 133, 199, 200
worms, 10, 20, 28, 43

Y

yeast, 21, 33, 34, 101, 107, 110
yield, 25, 205

W

Waterhouse-Friderichsen syndrome, 218, 223, 224

Z

zinc finger nucleases (ZFNs), x, 84, 86, 95, 97, 98, 99, 106
zygote, 89, 112